# Atlas of Intraoperative Cranial Nerve Monitoring in Thyroid and Head and Neck Surgery

Alexander L. Shifrin • Alan D. Deutsch
Gregory W. Randolph
Editors

# Atlas of Intraoperative Cranial Nerve Monitoring in Thyroid and Head and Neck Surgery

Springer

*Editors*
Alexander L. Shifrin
Surgical Director of Endocrinology
Atlantic Health CentraState Medical Center
Freehold, NJ, USA

Gregory W. Randolph
Otolaryngology Head and Neck Surgery
Claire and John Bertucci Endowed Chair in Thyroid Surgical Oncology
Harvard Medical School
Boston, MA, USA

Alan D. Deutsch
Monmouth Ocean Neurology
Neptune, NJ, USA

ISBN 978-3-031-24615-9 ISBN 978-3-031-24613-5 (eBook)
https://doi.org/10.1007/978-3-031-24613-5



This Springer imprint is published by the registered company Springer Nature Switzerland AG
The registered company address is: Gewerbestrasse 11, 6330 Cham, Switzerland

# Preface

The recurrent laryngeal nerve (RLN), the external branch of the superior laryngeal nerve (EBSLN), the vagus nerve, the spinal accessory nerve, the hypoglossal nerve, and the phrenic nerve can be at risk during thyroid, parathyroid, and modified radical neck dissection surgery.

The most common injury during thyroidectomy, injury to the RLN, can significantly impact the quality of life, altering the ability to speak, swallow, and/or breathe and may risk tracheotomy. Serious consequences also will result from injuries to the vagus, the hypoglossal, the spinal accessory, and the phrenic nerves.

Successful management and preservation of these nerves during thyroid, parathyroid, and radical modified neck dissection surgery requires a thorough understanding of the anatomy and function of nerves. Intraoperative neurophysiologic monitoring (IONM) has gained increased acceptance since its early description over 50 years ago as an adjunctive technique for nerves preservation, offering a dynamic functional assessment of the nerves' functions. Utilization of IONM enables the surgeon to interrogate nerve anatomy and function with immediate quantitative feedback, thereby augmenting surgical training. Importantly, surgical skills and sound anatomic knowledge remain prerequisites and are not supplanted by IONM use. Application of IONM in head and neck surgery, including indications, techniques, and pitfalls, is required for residents and fellows in surgery, specifically endocrine surgery and otolaryngology-head and neck surgery programs. For those receiving fellowship training under the supervision of the AHNS or the AAES, thorough understanding and ability to perform IONM of the RLN is required. As exposure to IONM during training has been shown to be associated with higher utilization by surgeons upon entering practice independently, continued increase in utilization is expected. Nonetheless, there remains inconsistency globally in training and application of IONM.

This Atlas is designed to help all endocrine surgeons, otolaryngology surgeons, and head and neck surgeons to learn the IONM technique, and to interpret the result of the nerves' stimulations, in order to prevent devastating injuries. This Atlas consists of several chapters that are specifically illustrating different nerves' responses and include the RLN, the EBSLN, the vagus nerve, the hypoglossal nerve, the spinal accessory nerve, and the phrenic nerve.

Freehold, NJ, USA — Alexander L. Shifrin
Neptune, NJ, USA — Alan D. Deutsch
Boston, MA, USA — Gregory W. Randolph

# Acknowledgments

The creation of this atlas was dependent on a team effort, which was possible only with the support and enthusiasm of the many individuals who contributed to this book: Hanna Kratochvil, Jeremy Goldfarb, Christopher Blake Sullivan, Erivelto Volpi, Joseph Scharpf, Amanda Silver Karcioglu, Marika D. Russell, Amr H. Abdelhamid Ahmed, Marcin Barczynski, Claudio R. Cernea, Joseph DiAngelo, Pedro Garcia, Thomas Lopazanski, Rick Schneider, Che-Wei Wu, Özer Makay, Gianlorenzo Donigi, and Amr H. Abdelhamid Ahmed who provided an additional support to numerous chapters in this Atlas. We thank our colleagues who trusted us and dedicated their time and effort to make it happen, without whom this Atlas would have never come to life!

Special thanks to Executive Editors Richard Hruska and Kristopher Spring, who believed in us, and Senior Editor Lee Klein of Springer for his hard work and dedication.

Finally, I would like to thank the entire staff at Springer, who were very supportive from the first idea of this atlas and maintained their enthusiasm throughout the project. Finally we wish to thank our patients with whom we learn the subtleties of surgical care of the neck base and their families who selflessly indulge us in this study.

# Contents

# Contributors

**Amr H. Abdelhamid Ahmed, MBBCH, MMSc, PGCert** Division of Thyroid and Parathyroid Endocrine Surgery, Department of Otolaryngology—Head and Neck Surgery, Massachusetts Eye and Ear Infirmary, Harvard Medical School, Boston, MA, USA

**Brittany Al-Atrache, MD** Jersey Shore University Medical Center, Neptune City, NJ, USA

**Marcin Barczyński, MD, PhD** Department of Endocrine Surgery, Third Chair of General Surgery, Jagiellonian University Medical College, Krakow, Poland

**Servet Celik, MD** Department of Anatomy, Faculty of Medicine, Ege University, Izmir, Turkey

**Claudio R. Cernea, MD, PhD** Department of Surgery, University of São Paulo School of Medicine, São Paulo, São Paulo, Brazil

**Alan D. Deutsch, DO** Monmouth Ocean Neurology, Neptune, NJ, USA

**Joseph DiAngelo, MD** Monmouth Ocean Neurology, Neptune, NJ, USA

**Gianlorenzo Dionigi, MD** Division of Surgery, Istituto Auxologico Italiano IRCCS (Istituto di Ricovero e Cura a Carattere Scientifco), Milan, Italy

**Francesco Frattini, MD** Division of General and Bariatric Surgery, Istituto Auxologico Italiano, IRCCS, Milan, Italy

**Pedro Garcia, MD** Monmouth Ocean Neurology, Neptune, NJ, USA

**Jeremy Goldfarb, MD** Massachusetts Eye and Ear, Inpatient Hospitalist Service, Harvard Medical School, Boston, MA, USA

**Amanda Silver Karcioglu, MD** Division of Otolaryngology—Head and Neck Surgery, Department of Surgery, NorthShore University HealthSystem, Evanston, IL, USA

The University of Chicago, Pritzker School of Medicine, Chicago, IL, USA

**Hanna Kratochvil, MD** Massachusetts Eye and Ear, Harvard Medical School, Boston, MA, USA

**Thomas Lopazanski, MD** Monmouth Ocean Neurology, Neptune, NJ, USA

**Özer Makay, MD** Department of General Surgery, Division of Endocrine Surgery, Ege University Hospital, Genel Cerrahi Kliniği, Izmir, Turkey

**Lawrence Mitelberg** Brooklyn College, Brooklyn, NY, USA

**Antonella Pino, MD** Division of Surgery, Istituto Auxologico Italiano IRCCS (Istituto di Ricovero e Cura a Carattere Scientifco), Milan, Italy

**Gregory W. Randolph, MD, FACS, FACE, FEBS (Endocrine)** Otolaryngology Head and Neck Surgery, Claire and John Bertucci Endowed Chair in Thyroid Surgical Oncology, Harvard Medical School, Boston, MA, USA

**Marika D. Russell, MD** Division of Thyroid and Parathyroid Endocrine Surgery, Department of Otolaryngology—Head and Neck Surgery, Massachusetts Eye and Ear Infirmary, Harvard Medical School, Boston, MA, USA

**Joseph Scharpf, MD, FACS** Head and Neck Institute, Cleveland Clinic Foundation, Cleveland, OH, USA

**Rick Schneider, MD** Department of Visceral, Vascular and Endocrine Surgery, University Hospital, Martin Luther University Halle-Wittenberg, Halle (Saale), Germany

**Alexander L. Shifrin, MD, FACS, FACE, ECNU, FEBS, FISS** Surgical Director of Endocrinology, Atlantic Health CentraState Medical Center, Freehold, NJ, USA

**Christopher Blake Sullivan, MD** Department of Otolaryngology—Head and Neck Surgery, University of North Carolina, Chapel Hill, NC, USA

**Erivelto Volpi, MD** Oncology Center of Hospital Alemao Oswaldo Cruz, Sao Paulo, Brazil

**Che-Wei Wu, MD, PhD** Department of Otorhinolaryngology-Head and Neck Surgery, Kaohsiung Medical University Hospital, Faculty of Medicine, College of Medicine, Kaohsiung Medical University, Kaohsiung, Taiwan

# Anatomy and Function of Cranial and Neck Nerves

1

Brittany Al-Atrache and Alexander L. Shifrin

## Introduction

This chapter describes the anatomy and function of the cranial nerves (CNs) and nerves of the neck, specifically emphasizing CNs that a surgeon would encounter during neck surgery, such as cranial nerve (CN) 5 with the marginal mandibular branch, CN X (vagus nerve), the recurrent laryngeal nerve (RLN), the superior laryngeal nerve (SLN), external branch of the superior laryngeal nerve (EBSLN), the Galen's anastomosis between the posterior branch of the internal laryngeal nerve and the recurrent laryngeal nerve, CN XI (spinal accessory nerve), and the CN XII (hypoglossal nerve). We also described anatomy and function of some non-cranial nerves of the neck, such as the phrenic nerve.

## Summary of Cranial Nerves I–VI, VII, and IX

Nuclei of CNs, except I and II, are located in the brainstem. They are divided into cisternal, intracranial, and extracranial segments. They are surrounded by connective tissue sheaths that are divided into endoneurium, perineurium, and epineurium segments from internal to external to the nerve [1].

## CNI: The Olfactory Nerve

CNI is a special afferent nerve for sense of smell function. CNI is part of the central nervous system pathway (in contrast to the other cranial nerves which have peripheral nervous system tracts). The olfactory system consists of olfactory epithelium, olfactory bulbs, olfactory striae and their target brain areas. Within the mucosa of the nasal cavity lie the olfactory receptors. The olfactory filiae or axons enter the anterior cranial fossa through the cribriform plate and terminate in the olfactory bulb [1]. Their cellular constituents are that of the CNS and therefore demonstrate CNS pathologies such as astrocytomas [2].

## CNII: The Optic Nerve

CNII is a special afferent nerve for vision. Similar to CNI, CNII is also part of the CNS pathway with central nervous system tracts. CN II is approximately 50 mm in length and is divided into four segments: intraocular, intraorbital, intracanalicular, and prechiasmatic [1]. The nerve is further divided into four quadrants based on location: superior/inferior and nasal/temporal. The flow of visual information begins with photoreceptors (composed of rods and cones containing light sensitive pigments), then is conducted to bipolar cells, and, finally, to ganglion cells. These signals are further modified by horizontal, amacrine and muller cells.

The optic chiasm is the area where the left and right optic nerves converge and the nasal fibers from each nerve decussate, while the temporal fibers do not [1]. Visual information from the retina is carried via the retinogeniculate pathway (primary pathway for visual information) to the lateral geniculate nucleus of the thalamus, the retinopretectal tract responsible for pupillary light reflex, retinocollicular tract to the superior colliculus responsible for eye movements, and the retinohypothalamic tract to the bilateral suprachiasmatic nuclei of the hypothalamus for circadian rhythms and endocrine function [2], and ultimately to the occipital lobes.

B. Al-Atrache
Jersey Shore University Medical Center, Neptune City, NJ, USA
e-mail: Brittany.Kane@hmhn.org

A. L. Shifrin (✉)
Surgical Director of Endocrinology, Atlantic Health CentraState Medical Center, Freehold, NJ, USA



A. L. Shifrin et al. (eds.), *Atlas of Intraoperative Cranial Nerve Monitoring in Thyroid and Head and Neck Surgery*,
https://doi.org/10.1007/978-3-031-24613-5_1

## CNIII: The Oculomotor Nerve

The oculomotor nerve has a somatic motor function for most of the ocular extrinsic muscles and a parasympathetic function to the ciliaris and sphincter pupillae muscles via the Edinger-Westphal nucleus. Somatic motor fibers originate from the nuclear complex at the level of the superior colliculus within the midbrain [1]. This provides somatic innervation to

1. Inferior rectus (IO): depresses eye
2. Superior rectus (SR): elevates eye
3. Medial rectus (MR): adducts eye
4. Inferior oblique (IO): elevates eye when eye adducted. Laterally rotates eye when eye abducted
5. Levator palpebrae superioris (LPS): raises eyelid

Subnuclei of this nerve supply the individual muscles. The lateral subnuclei supply the ipsilateral IR, IO, and MR muscles. Medial subnucleus supplies contralateral SR. Central subnucleus in the midline supplies the LPS bilaterally. The general visceral efferent provides parasympathetic innervation to:

1. Sphincter pupillae: Constricts pupil
2. Ciliary muscles: Contraction causes lens to bulge (accommodation) [2].

## CN IV: The Trochlear Nerve

The trochlear nerve is a general somatic efferent nerve providing somatic motor innervation to the superior oblique (SO) muscles. The trochlear nucleus lies inferior to the oculomotor nuclear complex within the inferior midbrain. The tendon of the SO muscle passes through the trochlea in the medial wall of the orbit and inserts on the sclera of the posterior lateral globe to act as a pulley. Contraction of the SO causes depression of the eye when the eye is adducted and inward rotation of the eye when the eye is abducted. The trochlear nerve is the smallest CN and has the longest intracranial course. Therefore, it may be directly visualized with only very high resolution MRI sequences or seen in cases of pathology [2].

## CN V: The Trigeminal Nerve

The trigeminal nerve is a general sensory afferent nerve and special visceral efferent nerve. The general sensory portion provides sensory input from skin and mucous membranes of face, forehead, anterior scalp, nasal/oral cavities, conjunctiva, paranasal sinuses, teeth, anterior two-thirds of tongue and part of the external surface of the tympanic membrane, dura of anterior and middle cranial fossae. The special visceral efferent portion innervates the muscles of mastication [2]. CNV leaves the midlateral surface of the pons as a large sensory root and a smaller anteromedial motor root at the cerebellopontine angle where it enters the subarachnoid space. It then enters Meckel's cave (a cerebrospinal fluid filled space between two layers of dura over the petrous portion of the temporal bone that encloses the trigeminal ganglion and all three roots of the trigeminal nerve) [1]. The three major divisions of the trigeminal nerve are:

V1—Ophthalmic
V2—Maxillary
V3—Mandibular

**V1** is a sensory branch of CNV. It enters the orbit through the superior orbital fissure (SOF) along with sensory nerves III, IV, and VI, sympathetic fibers from internal carotid artery plexus, superior ophthalmic vein, orbital branch of middle meningeal artery, and the recurrent meningeal branch of the lacrimal artery.

**V2** is a sensory branch of CNV. It gives off the middle meningeal nerve to innervate the dura of the middle cranial fossa. V2 runs with the emissary veins and the artery of foramen to exit the cranial vault via the foramen rotundum. It then further branches in the pterygopalatine fossa into the infraorbital nerve, zygomatic nerve, and other sensory nerve fibers to the orbital, palatine posterior superior nasal and pharyngeal branches.

**V3** involves both sensory and motor branches of CNV and is the largest of the three divisions. The sensory root of V3 lies in Meckel's Cave and, along with the lesser superficial petrosal nerve, emissary veins, and accessory meningeal artery, exits the skull via the foramen ovale. It then joins the motor root to form the mandibular nerve in the infratemporal fossa where it further divides into the meningeal branch, medial pterygoid nerve, masseteric nerve and deep temporal nerves, buccal nerve, lateral pterygoid nerve, auriculotemporal nerve, lingual nerve, and inferior alveolar nerve. The motor component of the mandibular nerve gives brachial motor innervation to the muscles of mastication [2].

## CN VI: The Abducens Nerve

CN VI provides general somatic efferent innervation to the lateral rectus (LR) muscle.

The abducens nucleus is located just beneath the floor of the IV ventricle in the dorsal pons [1]. It lies within the cavernous sinus adjacent to the ICA (unlike CN III, IV, V1, V2 which lie in the lateral wall of the cavernous sinus) to innervate the LR muscle to abduct the eye [2].

## CN IX: The Glossopharyngeal Nerve

CN IX is a mixed nerve with both motor, sensory and parasympathetic pathways arising from its nuclei. The four nuclei of CN IX are located within the medulla. They include the ambiguus nucleus, inferior salivary nucleus, spinal nucleus of the trigeminal nerve, and the solitary nucleus. CN IX exits the cranium within the jugular foramen where it gives off the tympanic nerve to supply parasympathetic innervation to the parotid gland [3]. As the nerve descends into the neck, it provides innervation to the stylopharyngeus and sensation to the carotid sinus and body. It then terminates in the pharynx between the superior and middle constrictors [4]. The most common injury to this nerve causes glossopharyngeal neuralgia (GPN) characterized by oropharyngeal pain triggered by swallowing, chewing, or yawning. The most common surgical procedure that can cause injury to this nerve is carotid endarterectomy. Transection of this nerve can present as glossopharyngeal nerve paresis which can result in dysphagia and dysphonia [5].

## CN VII: The Facial Nerve

### Anatomy

The nucleus of the facial motor nerve is anterolateral to the nucleus of CN VI within the caudal pontine tegmentum in the lower portion of the pons. Its axons travel around the nucleus of CN VI as part of the corticobulbar fibers and then progress ventrolateral to the pontomedullary junction. These fibers project to the upper face motor neurons and to the lower face motor neurons. The peripheral course of CN VII emanates from the ventrolateral pons and travels along the cerebellopontine angle cistern to enter the petrous portion of the temporal bone. Within this region, CN VII further divides into four segments: the meatal segment, the labyrinthine segment, the horizontal segment, and the mastoid segment [2].

The mastoid segment lies within the posterior middle ear to give off three branches: the nerve to the stapedius muscle, the chordae tympani, the sensory auricular branch that innervates the external auditory meatus and the auricular/retroauricular area.

The nerve then gives off the posterior auricular nerve as it exits the stylomastoid foramen. This branch innervates the occipitalis, posterior auricular and oblique auricular muscles. It further branches to form the digastric branch and the stylohyoid branch. CN VII then enters the parotid gland and divides into the temporal facial and cervicofacial branches. These branches further divide into the temporal, zygomatic, bucca, marginal mandibular and cervical branches to innervate the muscles of facial expression [2]. These nerves travel deep to the parotid masseteric fascia and lie above the deep cervical investing layer [4].

The marginal mandibular branch is at risk of injury during surgical procedures such as excision of the submandibular gland, parotidectomy, temporomandibular joint surgery, neck dissection, and thyroidectomy [4]. This nerve lies at the angle of the mandible and passes downward over the surface of the posterior facial vein. The marginal mandibular nerve has been found to run either superficial, deep, or both to the facial artery, most commonly lying anterior to the artery. The nerve can then run above the inferior border of the mandible or 1 cm or less below the inferior border of the mandible. Iatrogenic injury to this nerve can cause significant defects in cosmetic facial appearance, including paralysis of the depressor anguli oris and the depressor labii inferioris. This causes inversion and flattening of the ipsilateral lip and inhibits inferior lateral movement (inability to pull the lower lip down and to the side) causing an asymmetrical smile with elevation of the lower lip [6]. Although there has been debate for many years regarding the safe distance to make the submandibular incision and avoid injury to this nerve, incisions made 2 cm below the lower border of the mandible will avoid injury to this nerve in nearly all circumstances [7].

### Function

The facial nerve consists of two portions: the proper VII nerve (motor function) and the intermediate nerve (sensory and parasympathetic motor fibers) [1]. The motor pathway is further divided into branchiomotor to innervate the muscles of facial expression (orbicularis oculi, orbicularis oris, zygomaticus major, levator anguli oris, risorius, corrugator supercilii, and platysma), as well as the stapedius, stylohyoid and posterior belly of digastric.

CN VII has multiple visceral motor branches to innervate multiple structures within the head and neck region. The greater petrosal nerve is a branch of CN VII that provides parasympathetic innervation to the lacrimal gland, oral, and nasal mucosa. The chordae tympani is another branch of CN VII that provides innervation to the submandibular and sublingual glands. CN VII also provides somatic sensory innervation to the external auditory meatus, auricle and retroauricular area as well as special sensory from the anterior two-thirds of the tongue via the chordae tympani to provide taste sensation [2].

## CN X: The Vagus Nerve

### Anatomy

CN 10 is the most widely distributed of the cranial nerves. Vagus is Latin for "wandering" [8]. The vagus nerve originates at the lateral medulla from the base of the nucleus ambiguous and the dorsal nucleus of the vagus as eight to ten rootlets that then converge into a single trunk. It then enters the lateral cerebellomedullary cistern and exits the skull through the jugular foramen (pars vascularis) between the glossopharyngeal and accessory nerve [1]. Within the jugular foramen, it lies posteriorly along with CN XI. The superior portion of the ganglion is termed the "jugular ganglion" and contains sensory neurons.

As it exits the jugular foramen, it forms the inferior ganglion and contains visceral and special sensory information. The main trunk of the vagus nerve then dives into the neck within the carotid sheath to give off the recurrent laryngeal and superior cardiac branches. The vagus nerve then crosses over the subclavian artery on the right side and between the common carotid and subclavian arteries on the left to enter the thorax. It then gives off fibers to the pulmonary and esophageal plexuses. CN X enters the diaphragm anterior to the esophagus on the left side and posterior to the esophagus on the right side. It is responsible for innervation to the abdominal organs as the gastric branches, celiac branches, and hepatic nerve [2].

*The right RLN* is a branch of the vagus nerve that arises in front of the subclavian artery. It then travels upward behind the subclavian artery into the tracheoesophageal groove. *The left RLN* travels beneath the ligamentum arteriosum before ascending into the left tracheoesophageal groove. This nerve innervates all intrinsic laryngeal muscles except the cricothyroid, which, as previously stated, is supplied by the external ramus of the SLN [2].

## Function

The Vagus nerve has four pathways:

1. *The special visceral efferent brachial motor pathway* innervates striated muscles of the soft palate, pharynx, and larynx via the nucleus ambiguous in the medulla. This pathway is responsible for the "gag" reflex. Touching the wall of one side of the pharynx in a normal individual will elicit a bilateral response. The afferent limb is via the glossopharyngeal nerve and the efferent limb is via the vagus nerve [8].
2. *The general visceral motor pathway* provides secretomotor innervation to pharyngeal mucosa, laryngeal mucosa, and thoracic organs, esophageal, gastric, celiac, and hepatic plexi.
3. *The visceral sensory pathway* afferent signals are sent from the pharynx, larynx, trachea, lungs, heart, alimentary tract (esophagus, stomach down to splenic flexure), aortic arch baroreceptors, and aortic body chemoreceptors to the inferior ganglion to the tractus solitarius and caudal nucleus solitarius.
4. *The special sensory pathway* of the vagus nerve provides taste information from the epiglottis, hard and soft palates, and pharynx to the inferior ganglion to the rostral nucleus solitarius. The nucleus solitarius has multiple nuclei, each with specific function. The rostral nucleus solitarius provides gustatory input. The caudal nucleus solitarius provides visceral sensation. The efferent fibers to thalamic ventral posteromedial nucleus and salivatory nucleus for salvation and taste and dorsal motor nucleus for increased peristalsis.

Vagal input from the aortic arch chemoreceptors synapse in the medullary respiratory center in response to $CO_2$ levels within the blood [2].

## Branches of the Vagus Nerve

There are two important branches of the vagus nerve: the superior laryngeal nerve (SLN) and the recurrent laryngeal nerve (RLN). Arising from the inferior ganglion of the vagus nerve, *the superior laryngeal nerve* travels down the side of the pharynx and divides into the external and internal laryngeal nerves. *The external branch of the superior laryngeal nerve* (EBSLN) supplies the inferior pharyngeal constrictor and cricothyroid muscles. *The internal branch of the superior laryngeal nerve* travels through the thyrohyoid membrane with the superior laryngeal nerve and sends sensory fibers to the epiglottis and mucous membranes of the larynx above the vocal cords.

### The Recurrent Laryngeal Nerve (RLN)

The RLN branches off the vagus nerve to supply all intrinsic muscles of the larynx except the cricothyroid muscle (Fig. 1.1). The right RLN branches at the level of T1-T2 and loops under the right subclavian artery. It then travels posteriorly and ascends in the posterior neck. The left RLN loops posteriorly under the aortic arch to travel back superiorly through the neck [9]. Damage to this nerve anywhere along its path can cause impaired vocal function. This occurs most commonly during surgical intervention, most frequently thyroidectomies and parathyroidectomies, accounting for nearly 30–40% of injuries. Injury to this nerve will present as new onset hoarseness or changes in vocal pitch secondary to vocal cord paralysis. Bilateral vocal cord paralysis, although less common, presents with much more serious symptoms. These include significant difficulties breathing and swallowing. Although recent neck surgery or recent intubation can cause injury to this structure, underlying malignancy including lymphadenopathy, thyroid masses, and lung apex tumors must be considered.

The RLN travels from the cranium to the thorax; therefore, imaging should involve any or all of these areas [10]. Evalu-

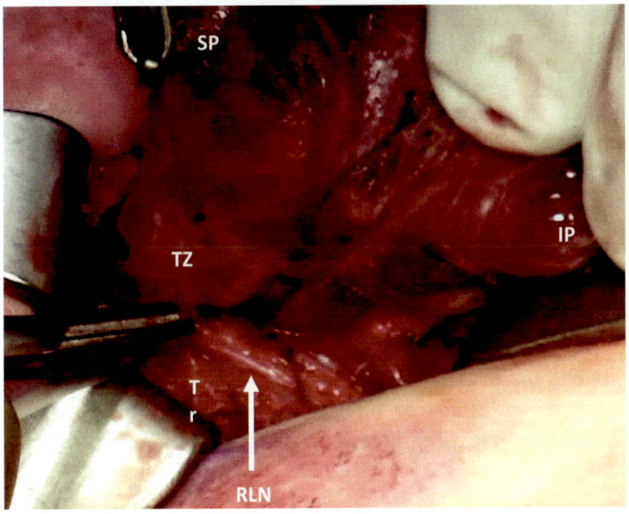


**Fig. 1.1** Normal anatomy of the recurrent laryngeal nerve (RLN) on the right side. The right RLN is usually positioned more obliquely and laterally to the tracheoesophageal groove compared to the left RLN. Left side of the screen—cephalad; right side of the screen—caudal. Arrow is pointing at the recurrent laryngeal nerve (RLN). *Tr* trachea, *SP* superior pole of the right thyroid lobe, *IP* inferior pole of the right thyroid lobe, *TZ* tubercle of Zuckerkandl

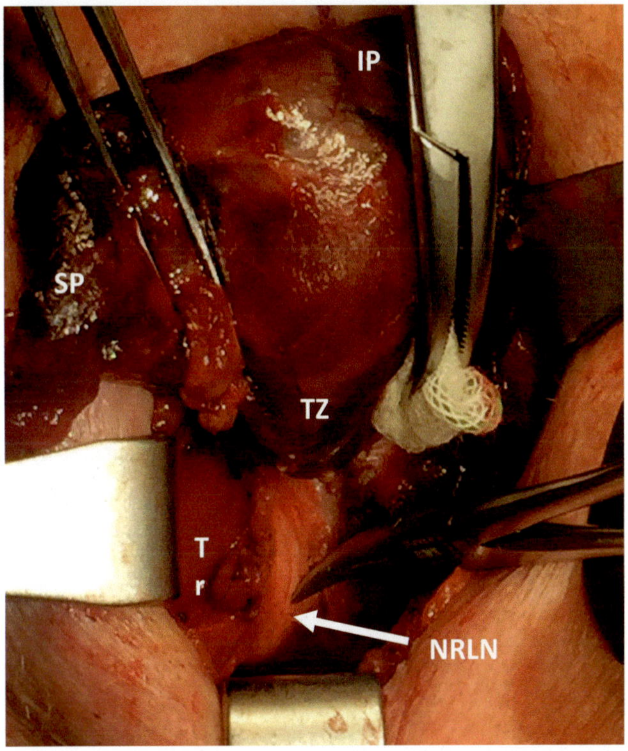


**Fig. 1.2** The non-recurrent laryngeal nerve (NRLN) on the right side. The RLN is seen as the non-recurrent (NRLN) coming off the vagus nerve from the carotid sheath laterally toward the cricothyroid muscle (arrow) rather than from the inferior direction as in Fig. 1.1. Left side of the screen—cephalad; right side of the screen—caudal. Arrow and mosquito are pointing at the non-recurrent laryngeal nerve (NRLN). *Tr* trachea, *SP* superior pole of the right thyroid lobe, *LP* inferior pole of the right thyroid lobe, *TZ* tubercle of Zuckerkandl

ation with CT scan is the most commonly used diagnostic modality because it images the nerve along its entire course. However, when patients present with vocal cord paralysis, direct laryngoscopy should be considered before CT [11].

Identifying the RLN is the gold standard for preventing injury during thyroid surgery [12, 13]. However, the RLN can have great anatomic variability and sometimes can have early division of its branches. In a difficult neck dissection, surgeons may change their dissection site or use an intraoperative neurostimulator [14].

The RLN may have anatomical variations in position and location of the right and the left RLNs. The right RLN (Fig. 1.1) comes off the main trunk of the right vagus nerve on the level of the right subclavian artery, hooks around the artery, and ascends up into the neck to enter into the cricothyroid muscle. The right RLN is usually positioned more obliquely and laterally to tracheoesophageal groove compared to the left RLN [15, 16]. The non-recurrent laryngeal nerve (NRLN) on the right side occurs in about 1% of patients (Fig. 1.2). In this case, the NRLN comes directly from the vagus nerve laterally at the level of the cricothyroid muscle and goes directly transverse to enter the cricothyroid muscle from the lateral location, rather than inferiorly. If the NRLN is not recognized, it can be easily injured. In the majority of cases, the presence of the NRLN associates with an aberrant right subclavian artery [6, 17].

The RLN can have up to six branches [16]. Bifurcation of the RLN was reported on the right side in between 26% and 33% of cases, and on the left side in 19–23% of cases, with bilateral bifurcation reported in about 8.9% of patients. The RLN bifurcates into two branches in about 70% of cases on the right side and 67% of cases on the left, and more than two branches in about 30% of cases on the right side and 33% of cases on the left side (Fig. 1.3). It is important to dissect the entire length of the neck part of the RLN during the thyroidectomy since it can bifurcate at more than 2 cm inferior to the larynx in 33% of patients on the right side, and 58% of cases on the left side. The most important anatomical considerations are given to the functional aspect of the RLN. The vocal cords' adduction and abduction is controlled exclusively by motor fibers located in the anterior (the more medial) branch of RLN, and none is present in the posterior (or lateral) branch(es) of the RLN. That is the reason why the exposure of the entire RLN during a surgical dissection is required in order to detect all branches of the nerve. Intraoperative monitoring of the RLN can help with nerve identification, mapping, and evaluation of function. Intraoperative RLN monitoring (IONM) is especially helpful with the branching nerve. Losing the IONM signal on one side of the RLN during dissection can influence the surgeon's decision to proceed to the other side with a total thyroidectomy [15, 18].

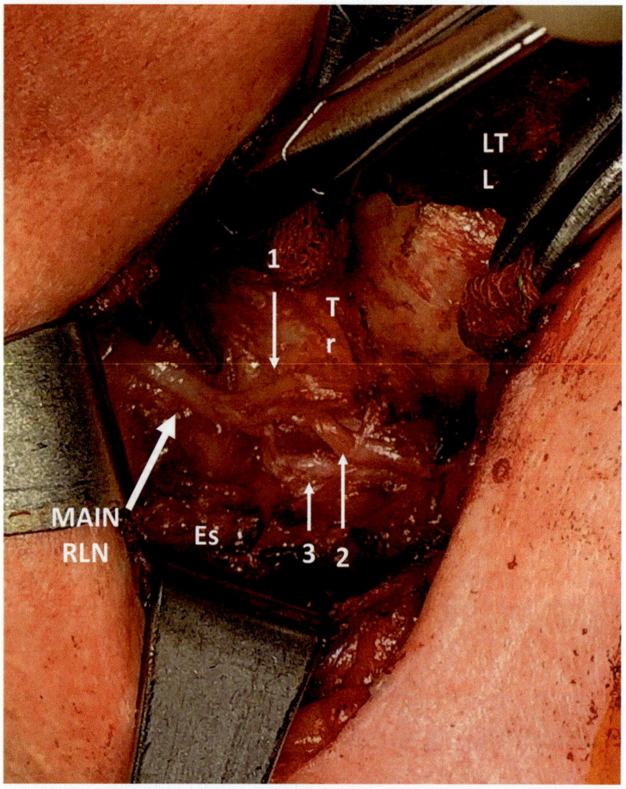


**Fig. 1.3** Bifurcation of the left RLN into three branches (arrows 1, 2, and 3). The vocal branch is the most medial and anterior branch (arrow 1). *LTL* left thyroid lobe, *Tr* trachea, *Es* esophagus, *MAIN RLN* the main trunk of the RLN; arrows 1, 2, and 3 are pointing to three branches of the left RLN

The anatomical relationship between the position of the inferior thyroid artery (ITA) and the RLN may vary. Most commonly, the RLN runs posterior to the ITA in about 76% of patients on both sides, anterior to the ITA in 19% of patients on the right side and 24% of patients on the left side, and in between the branches of the RLN in about 3.3% of patients on the right side and less than that on the left side [17, 19]. If the RLN runs in between the branches of the ITA, retracting the thyroid lobe up and medially may cause pressure from one of the ITA branches causing "strangulation injury" of the RLN and may result in transient neural paralysis.

## Superior Laryngeal Nerve (SLN)

The superior laryngeal nerve originates from the vagus nerve at the level of C2 vertebra and travels inferiorly and medially toward the thyrohyoid membrane (TM) which lies between the thyroid cartilage and hyoid bone [20]. The SLN may be injured during anterior or anterolateral cervical spine surgery, thyroid surgery, or carotid endarterectomy. Injury to this nerve causes impairment of the laryngeal cough reflex. Patient's with injury to this nerve may be at greater risk for aspiration pneumonia or other respiratory illnesses [20].

To prevent injury to this nerve, understanding of the anatomy of the region of the superior thyroid pole and the superior laryngeal nerve is crucial. Careful exposure and independent ligation of the superior thyroid artery branches close to the thyroid capsule are necessary to avoid injury to this nerve. Neuromodulating can also be helpful; however, visual identification of the nerve, although useful, is not always possible [21].

The SLN divides into the *internal* and *external* branches close to the internal carotid artery.

### The Internal Branch of the Superior Laryngeal Nerve (IBSLN)

*The internal branch of the superior laryngeal nerve* (IBSLN) is accompanied by the superior laryngeal artery passing inferiorly to the greater horn of the hyoid bone and travels toward the TM. The IBSLN is further divided into three branches: the superior branch, which innervates the mucosa of the epiglottis and a small part of the anterior wall of the vallecula; the middle branch, which contains sensory fibers and innervates the aryepiglottic folds; and the interior branch, which supplies a portion of the interarytenoid muscles [20]. In 72.22% of cases the IBSLN divides into three branches and in 27.78% of cases it divides into two branches prior to penetration into the thyrohyoid membrane [22]. The IBSLN contains afferents nerve fibers coming from the supraglottic larynx and epiglottis. The function of the IBSLN includes: laryngeal closure, induction of swallowing movements, central apnea, and strong resetting of the respiratory rhythm [23].

### The External Branch of the Superior Laryngeal Nerve (EBSLN)

*The external branch of the superior laryngeal nerve* (EBSLN) is the only motor supply to the cricothyroid muscle [24] (Fig. 1.4). The EBSLN runs through the sternothyroid-laryngeal triangle defined by Moosman and De Weese in 1968 [25]. There is a significant variation in the course of the EBSLN resulting in the high incidence of injury to this nerve. Cernea, CR developed the classification for the anatomical position of the EBSL in relation to the superior pole of the thyroid lobe (*see* Fig. 6.2). Type 1—nerve is crossing the superior thyroid vessels 1 or more cm above a horizontal plane passing the upper border of the superior thyroid pole, in 60% of patients. Type 2—nerve is crossing the vessels less than 1 cm above or below that horizontal plane: Type 2a—nerve is crossing less than 1 cm above the plane, in 17% of patients; Type 2b—nerve is crossing below the plane, in 20% of patients. Approximately in 3% of patients, the EBSLN has not been identified [26].

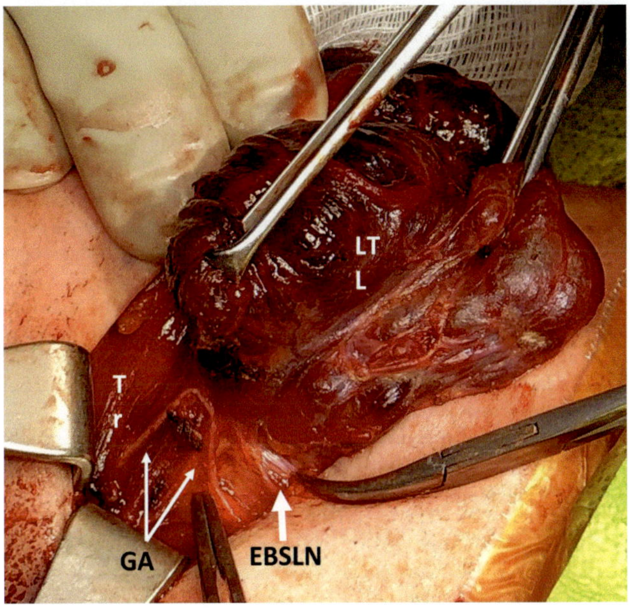


**Fig. 1.4** The external branch of the superior laryngeal nerve (EBSLN) and the Galen's anastomosis. *LTL* left thyroid lobe, *Tr* trachea, *EBSLN* the external branch of the superior laryngeal nerve, *GA* the Galen's anastomosis

Function of the EBSLN is very important during phonation and comes into play at frequencies above 150 Hz. The EBSLN is particularly involved in the production of high tones of the female voice range. It controls the frequency of vibration of the vocal cords that depends on the size, shape, and elastic tension of the vocal folds. For "chest tone" the cords assume rounded, full shape, and relaxed position; and for "falsetto tone" the cords assume sharp edged, thin, and taut shape. In addition, a degree of fine tuning of the voice is achieved by contraction of the vocalis muscle (the medial fibers of the thyroarytenoid), which is supplied by the recurrent laryngeal nerve [27].

## Communicating "Anastomoses" Between SLN and RLN

There are at least four anastomoses described between the IBSLN and the RLN: (1) Galen's anastomosis, a connection between the dorsal branches of both nerves; (2) arytenoid plexus, a connection between the arytenoid branches of both nerves; (3) cricoid anastomosis, in the front of the cricoid lamina; and (4) thyroarytenoid anastomosis, a connection of a descending branch of the IBSLN and an ascending branch of the RLN [28, 29].

An anastomosis between the IBSLN and the EBSLN appeared as a connecting branch throughout the foramen thyroideum [29].

An anastomosis between the EBSLN and the RLN appeared as a connecting branch throughout the cricothyroid muscle per Sañudo [29], or "cricothyroid connection" occurs in the piriform fossa [28].

## Galen's Anastomosis

The Galen's anastomosis is the direct connection between the posterior branch of the internal laryngeal nerve and the recurrent laryngeal nerve and that is located over the posterior surface of the posterior cricoarytenoid, transverse and oblique arytenoid muscles under the mucosa of the hypopharynx [28] (Fig. 1.4).

## Extra-Laryngeal Anastomosis Between the RLN and the EBSLN

Extra-laryngeal anastomosis between the RLN and the EBSLN has been identified in about 3% of patients [26].

## CN XI: The Spinal Accessory Nerve

The spinal accessory nerve is a purely motor CN. It is responsible for general somatic efferent motor innervation of the trapezius and sternocleidomastoid muscles. Cervical levels C1 through C5/C6 contain the spinal nucleus of the accessory nerve. These fibers enter the cranial vault via the foramen magnum and exit via the jugular foramen. Damage to this nerve causes ipsilateral flaccid paralysis of the sternocleidomastoid and shoulder drop secondary to paralysis of the trapezius muscle. Flaccid paralysis is not seen with the trapezius muscle due to the dual innervation by the anterior horn gray matter from C3 through C5/C6 [30].

## CN XII: The Hypoglossal Nerve

The hypoglossal nerve is also a pure motor CN. It is responsible for general somatic efferent innervation of all intrinsic and extrinsic muscles of the tongue except the palatoglossus muscle. Fibers from this nerve come together to exit the cranium between the pyramids and olives within the medulla. Damage to this nerve results in tongue deviation toward the side of the lesion as the weak or flaccid ipsilateral genioglossus muscle cannot overcome the opposing muscular force from the contralateral intact musculature [31].

## Phrenic Nerve

The phrenic nerve originates from the anterior rami of the C3 through C5 nerve roots and consists of motor, sensory, and sympathetic nerve fibers [32]. There are also accessory fibers originating from the subclavian nerve, the ansa cervicalis, and the sternohyoid nerve that join the phrenic nerve [33]. In 1853 Luschka described communicating fibers between the sympathetic trunk and the phrenic nerve in the cervical region. The phrenicoabdominal branch is a continuation of the right phrenic nerve toward the aortic autonomic plexus in the abdomen [33]. After originating from the cervical plexus, the phrenic nerve travels in the posterior triangle of the neck. The posterior triangle is defined by the sternocleidomastoid muscle, trapezius, and clavicle. Then the nerve descends to the anterior surface of the anterior scalene muscle obliquely from the posterior margin to the anterior. The phrenic nerve crosses the anterior border of the anterior scalene muscle at approximately Erb's point and then enters the thorax by passing in front of the subclavian artery [34, 35]. The phrenic nerve is the motor nerve to the diaphragm with sensory supply to the peripheral part of the diaphragm. Injury to the phrenic nerve will result in paralysis of the diaphragm.

## References


1. Romano N, Federici M, Castaldi A. Imaging of cranial nerves: a pictorial overview. Insights Imaging. 2019;10:33.
2. Binder DK, Sonne C, Fischbein NJ. Cranial nerves: anatomy, pathology, imaging. Thieme Medical Publishers; 2010.
3. Singh O, Das JM. StatPearls [Internet]. In: Anatomy, head and neck, jugular foramen. Treasure Island, FL: StatPearls Publishing; 2021.
4. Sindel A, Ozalp O, Yildirimyan N, Oguz N, Sindel M, Llankovan V. Evaluation of the course of the marginal mandibular branch of the facial nerve: a fresh cadaveric study. Br J Oral Maxillofac Surg. 2021;59(2):179–83.
5. Voskanian IE, Kolomeĭtsev SN, Shniukov RV. Risk factors and prevention of injuries to the cranial nerves in reconstructive surgery of the carotid arteries. Angiol Sosud Khir. 2005;11(2):96–103.
6. Dimonge JA, Basnayaka MODB, Yasith M, Ajith PM. Preserving the marginal mandibular branch of the facial nerve during submandibular region surgery: a cadaveric safety study. Patient Saf Surg. 2018;12:23.
7. Nason RW, Binahmed A, Torchia MG, Thliversis J. Clinical observation of the anatomy and function of the marginal mandibular nerve. Int J Oral Maxillofac Surg. 2007;36(8):712–5.
8. Vanderah TW, Gould DJ. Cranial nerves and their nuclei. In: Nolte's the human brain, vol. 12; 2020. p. 286–308.
9. Hlaller JM, Iwanik M, Shen FH. Clinically relevant anatomy of recurrent laryngeal nerve. Spine. 2012;37(2):97–100.
10. Paquette CM, Manos DC, Psooy BJ. Unilateral vocal cord paralysis: a review of CT findings, mediastinal causes, and the course of the recurrent laryngeal nerves. Radiographics. 2012;32(3):721–40.
11. Estes C, Sadoughi B, Mauer E, Christos P, Sulica L. Laryngoscopic and stroboscopic signs in the diagnosis of vocal fold paresis. Laryngoscope. 2017;127(9):2100–5.
12. Randolph GW, Kamani D. Intraoperative electrophysiologic monitoring of the recurrent laryngeal nerve during thyroid and parathyroid surgery: experience with 1,381 nerves at risk. Laryngoscope. 2017;127(1):280–6.
13. Steurer M, Passler C, Denk DM, et al. Advantages of recurrent laryngeal nerve identification in thyroidectomy and parathyroidectomy and the importance of preoperative and postoperative laryngoscopic examination in more than 1000 nerves at risk. Laryngoscope. 2002;112:124–33.
14. Page C, Cuvelier P, Biet A, et al. Value of intra-operative neuromonitoring of the recurrent laryngeal nerve in total thyroidectomy for benign goitre. J Laryngol Otol. 2015;129:553–7.
15. Randolph GW. The recurrent and superior laryngeal nerves. New York: Springer; 2016.
16. Rustad WH. The recurrent laryngeal nerves in thyroid surgery hardcover. Thomas; 1956.
17. Randolph GW. Surgery of the thyroid and parathyroid glands. 2nd ed. Philadelphia: Elsevier; 2012.
18. Donatini G, Carnaille B, Dionigi G. Increased detection of nonrecurrent inferior laryngeal nerve (NRLN) during thyroid surgery using systematic intraoperative nerve monitoring (IONM). World J Surg. 2013;37(1):91–3.
19. Wojtczak B, Kaliszewski K, Sutkowski K, Bolanowski M, Barczyński M. A functional assessment of anatomical variants of the recurrent laryngeal nerve during thyroidectomies using nerve monitoring. Endocrine. 2018;59(1):82–9.
20. Kiray A, Naderi S, Ergur I, Korman E. Surgical anatomy of the internal branch of the superior laryngeal nerve. Eur Spine J. 2006;15(9):1320–5.
21. Markogiannakis H, Zografos GC, Manouras A. Prevention of superior laryngeal nerve injury in thyroid surgery. Hell J Surg. 2015;87(1):85–55.
22. Paraskevas GK, Raikos A, Ioannidis O, Brand-Saberi B. Topographic anatomy of the internal laryngeal nerve: surgical considerations. Head Neck. 2012;34(4):534–40. https://doi.org/10.1002/hed.21769. Epub 2011 Apr 26. PMID: 21523845.
23. Jafari S, Prince RA, Kim DY, Paydarfar D. Sensory regulation of swallowing and airway protection: a role for the internal superior laryngeal nerve in humans. J Physiol. 2003;550(Pt 1):287–304. https://doi.org/10.1113/jphysiol.2003.039966.
24. Sakorafas GH, Kokoropoulos P, Lappas C, Sampanis D, Smyrniotis V. External branch of the superior laryngeal nerve: applied surgical anatomy and implications in thyroid surgery. Am Surg. 2012;78(9):986–91. PMID: 22964209.
25. Moosman DA, DeWeese MS. The external laryngeal nerve is related to thyroidectomy. Surg Gynecol Obstet. 1968;127(5):1011–6. PMID: 5681348.
26. Cernea CR, Ferraz AR, Nishio S, Dutra A Jr, Hojaij FC, Dos Santos LRM. Surgical anatomy of the external branch of the superior laryngeal nerve. Head Neck. 1992;14:380–3. https://doi.org/10.1002/hed.2880140507.
27. Kark AE, Kissin MW, Auerbach R, Meikle M. Voice changes after thyroidectomy: role of the external laryngeal nerve. Br Med J (Clin Res Ed). 1984;289(6456):1412–5. https://doi.org/10.1136/bmj.289.6456.1412.
28. Naidu L, Lazarus L, Partab P, Satyapal KS. Laryngeal nerve "anastomoses". Folia Morphol (Warsz). 2014;73(1):30–6. https://doi.org/10.5603/FM.2014.0005.

29. Sañudo JR, Maranillo E, León X, Mirapeix RM, Orús C, Quer M. An anatomical study of anastomoses between the laryngeal nerves. Laryngoscope. 1999;109(6):983–7. https://doi.org/10.1097/00005537-199906000-00026. PMID: 10369294.
30. Wiater JM, Bigliani LU. Spinal accessory nerve injury. Clin Orthop Relat Res. 1999;368:5–16.
31. Sonne J, Reddy V, Lopez-Ojeda W. StatPearls {Internet}. In: Neuroanatomy, cranial nerve. Treasure Island, FL: StatPearls Publishing; 2021.
32. Oliver KA, Ashurst JV. Anatomy, thorax, phrenic nerves. [Updated 2021 July 26]. In: StatPearls [Internet]. Treasure Island, FL: StatPearls Publishing; 2022. Available from: https://www.ncbi.nlm.nih.gov/books/NBK513325/.
33. Verlinden TJM, van Dijk P, Herrler A, et al. The human phrenic nerve serves as a morphological conduit for autonomic nerves and innervates the caval body of the diaphragm. Sci Rep. 2018;8:11697.
34. Hamada T, Usami A, Kishi A, et al. Anatomical study of phrenic nerve course in relation to neck dissection. Surg Radiol Anat. 2015;37:255–8. https://doi.org/10.1007/s00276-014-1343-1.
35. Standring S, Berkovitz KB, Shah P, et al. Neck and diaphragm and phrenic nerve. In: Gray's anatomy. 39th ed. Elsevier, Churchill Livingstone; 2004, pp. 534, 1084.

# 2 Electrophysiological Equipment

Lawrence Mitelberg and Alexander L. Shifrin

Assessment of cranial nerve functions are essential during head and neck surgeries in order to avoid complications that could be life threatening. Different neuromonitoring equipment has been designed to assist the surgeon during surgical procedures and to avoid irreversible damage. There are several different companies that are manufacturing equipment for neuromonitoring used during head and neck surgery, and especially for the monitoring of the recurrent laryngeal nerve (RLN) during the thyroid surgery [1–4].

## Medtronic

### NIM 3.0 System

NIM 3.0 system [5], designed by Medtronic, has two versions of NIM 3.0: NIM-Response 3.0 and NIM-Neuro 3.0. The benefits of both devices are the ability to collect data easily, real-time monitoring, and real-time warning if any nerves are injured during the procedure. While both devices assist in neuromonitoring, they have their differences such as the number of channels that can be used. The NIM-Response 3.0 can use up to 4 channels, while the NIM-Neuro 3.0 can use up to 8 channels for monitoring. The NIM- Neuro 3.0 is used for surgeries that have a higher risk factor for injuries, such as glomus or acoustic tumor removals. The NIM-Response 3.0 is more commonly used for ear, nose, and throat (ENT) surgeries. The NIM-Neuro 3.0 has an additional microscope overlay, while the surgeon operates on the patient.

The NIM 3.0 works by placing electrodes on the patient, which is an easy process because the device has a color-coded visual showing where the electrodes should be placed. When activated and working, the electrodes monitor an electromyographic (EMG) and then give audio and visual feedback to the surgeon (or the staff operator) on whether or not there is a disturbance to the nerve. In order to get further increase in accuracy and precision in the monitoring, monopolar and bipolar simulating probes and dissecting instruments are available that cooperate with the NIM 3.0 system.

### NIM Vital

The NIM Vital is another system designed by Medtronic that provides the surgeon with a live view of an EMG response from the electrodes placed on the muscle that will give off direct signals to the system. The electrodes are placed on color-coded placement guides and will visually and audibly notify the surgeon or the staff member if the nerve is being injured during the procedure.

The NIM Vital features a noise suppression system that will help to avoid noises from the surrounding equipment that may interfere with the system. This device is wireless; therefore, it can be placed at any part of the operation room and avoid additional hazard from tripping over multiple connecting wires. The user-friendly interface makes it easy to understand how the system functions with the ability of adding future characteristics to the system.

### NIM TriVantage EMG Tubes

The NIM TriVantage is another Medtronic system that is used during a thyroidectomy and neck surgery that is designed to monitor the RLN and the vagus nerve in order to prevent damage and unintended manipulation. The NIM TriVantage includes different standard size endotracheal tubes that are non-reinforced, and DEHP-free PVC with silver ink EMG electrodes. Endotracheal tube electrodes position over the vocal cords. The endotracheal tubes work with

L. Mitelberg
Brooklyn College, Brooklyn, NY, USA

A. L. Shifrin (✉)
Surgical Director of Endocrinology, Atlantic Health CentraState Medical Center, Freehold, NJ, USA



A. L. Shifrin et al. (eds.), *Atlas of Intraoperative Cranial Nerve Monitoring in Thyroid and Head and Neck Surgery*,
https://doi.org/10.1007/978-3-031-24613-5_2

the NIM 3.0 and NIM Vital to provide the operator with accurate information regarding the RNL of vagal nerve function [2–4].

## Inomed

### C2 Explore

C2 Explore [6], manufactured by Inomed, is designed to monitor the RLN during surgery. It uses advanced laryngeal monitoring (ALM) which enhances the signal recording by using eight sensor pads that permit 360° surface sensor coverage which is then transferred into 4 different channels. Then, the one with the best signals is displayed on the monitor. The monitor itself has a large display with acoustic signals eliminating a loss of signal. It is easy to learn and to read the data being displayed. It has the ability to export any of the data taken intraoperatively, even after a long period of time. There is a built-in LED scanner that can read QR codes which may contain patient data. The device has a built-in gesture Controle function to facilitate touchless manipulation.

## Cadwell

### Cascade IOMAX

The Cascade IOMAX, manufactured by Cadwell, can be used for different types of head and neck (ENT) and neurosurgery procedures. The equipment is designed to withstand any water damage, as well as mechanical damage to the device. There are six pieces of this equipment that compose the system:

- The IOMAX Cortical module: This module monitors the patient's cerebral functions with the ability to connect four limb modules.
- IOMAX Base Module: The power source for all the equipment.
- The IOMAX Limb Module: This module monitors the motor function of the patient's extremities during surgery.
- The New IONMAX 32-Channel Amplifier: Records EEG and SSEPs.
- LCSwap: A switch for direct cortical stimulation.

### CadX

CadX, by Cadwell, is designed to predict what will happen during surgery, specifically the technical and surgical effects of a surgery. The CadX allows the surgeon to simulate IONM data. The CadX provides the surgeon with case scenarios that show a surgical outcome. The device simulates anesthesia, technical setup, trace characteristics, surgical effects, pedicle screw, and scripts [1]. The device is user-friendly and if needed will teach the user how to properly and effectively use the equipment.

### Cascade Surgical Studio (CSS)

CSS is a program that allows the patient's IONM waveforms to be directly transcribed to the doctor. The system gives live visuals of the workflow and gives the ability to capture and save the visuals being displayed on the monitor. During a procedure to have references of previously saved data, the operator will be able to have the ability to see the live view of the IONM and the saved data/images of IONM. While the system is working, the staff will be able to monitor several different modalities in the operating room, through many different open windows on the screen with multi-channel settings.

## References


1. Cascade Surgical Studio. Cadwell. n.d.. Retrieved from https://www.cadwell.com/cascade_ionm_software/.
2. Chiang FY, Lu IC, Chen HC, Chen HY, Tsai CJ, Hsiao PJ, et al. Anatomical variations of recurrent laryngeal nerve during thyroid surgery: how to identify and handle the variations with intraoperative neuromonitoring. Kaohsiung J Med Sci. 2010;26(11):575–83. https://doi.org/10.1016/S1607-551X(10)70089-9.
3. Choi SY, Son YI. Intraoperative neuromonitoring for thyroid surgery: the proven benefits and limitations. Clin Exp Otorhinolaryngol. 2019;12(4):335–6. https://doi.org/10.21053/ceo.2019.00542.
4. Ghatol D, Widrich J. Intraoperative neurophysiological monitoring. [Updated 2022 May 8]. In: StatPearls [Internet]. Treasure Island, FL: StatPearls Publishing; 2022. Available from: https://www.ncbi.nlm.nih.gov/books/NBK563203/.
5. https://www.medtronic.com/us-en/healthcare-professionals/products/ear-nose-throat/neuromonitoring/nerveintegrity-monitor-3.html.
6. https://www.en.inomed.com/products/intraoperative-neuromonitoring-ionm/c2-xplore/.

# Intraoperative Neurophysiologic Monitoring: A Neurologic Perspective

3

Alan D. Deutsch

Intraoperative neurophysiologic monitoring (IONM) is the technique whereby vital neurologic structures that could potentially be placed in harm's way during the course of a surgical procedure are observed and closely followed for any signal changes. Neural structures elicit electrical potentials which with modern electrical equipment and computers amplify these signals such that they can be visualized and heard acoustically. Over the past several decades, great strides have been made in the field of IONM. Beginning with only somatosensory evoked potential monitoring for spinal surgery, the field has blossomed into a multi-modality approach for monitoring of various central nervous system tracts and peripheral nerve processes during a variety of surgeries to best protect all neural structures at possible risk during a particular surgery.

Through a variety of various electrophysiologic techniques of intraoperative monitoring including electroencephalography (EEG), somatosensory evoked potentials (SSEP), motor evoked potentials (MEP), brainstem auditory evoked responses (BAER), spinal D and I wave monitoring, free running continuous electromyography (EMG), stimulus triggered EMG, pedicle screw stimulation, cortical mapping, direct cortical stimulation, etc., different eloquent neuroanatomic structures can have their electrical integrity assessed through the use of baseline preoperative, intraoperative, and postoperative recordings. Electrical changes can be utilized to predict potential harm to a particular neural structure or structures that may be placed in harm's way during surgery either by compression, traction, ischemia, transection, etc. and inform the surgeon early in order to avoid permanent neurologic injury. A reduction in amplitude of a response (MEP or SSEP), complete loss of a response, prolongation in latency of a response, the need for an increase in stimulation intensity from baseline, focal slowing on continuous EEG, absence of a triggered response on EMG, or neurotonic discharges on free running continuous EMG may each serve to warn of potential injury to a particular structure or neurologic pathway being monitored in the area where the surgeon may be operating and allow for appropriate surgical measures to avoid permanent neurologic deficits.

The IONM team in the operating room consists of the surgeon, the anesthesiologist, the IONM technician, and the neurophysiologist. Each has their part to play as a member of the team. All rely on each other to best protect the safety of patients throughout their surgical procedure. The surgeon with their knowledge of anatomy can predict which neurologic structures may be jeopardized during a particular surgical procedure and as such inform the technician and neurophysiologist which neurologic structures could potentially be injured, which then dictates which modalities would be best to monitor in order to best protect these neurologic structures during the course of surgery. The anesthesiologist must choose the correct anesthetic agents and concentrations for induction and maintenance anesthesia to ensure adequate anesthesia, yet allow for recording of various neurophysiologic responses that may be negatively influenced by a particular anesthetic agent or their concentration. Blood pressure, heart rate, and temperature changes may also affect neurophysiologic signals and monitoring these are vital as well. The IONM technician is responsible for connecting the patient safely to the recording and stimulating equipment with various appropriate electrodes, wires, cables, etc. to ensure adequate recording and documentation of neurophysiologic signals and responses throughout the surgery. Documentation of anesthesia, vital signs, the steps within a surgical procedure as the case proceeds, and recording and storing of responses by the IONM Technician all serve to assist the neurophysiologist in order to best monitor and interpret responses throughout the surgery. Constant real-time monitoring of responses, the ability to interpret electrical changes and relay this information immediately to the surgeon and monitoring team, and troubleshooting any technical problems are the job of the neurophysiologist.

A. D. Deutsch (✉)
Monmouth Ocean Neurology, Neptune, NJ, USA


A. L. Shifrin et al. (eds.), *Atlas of Intraoperative Cranial Nerve Monitoring in Thyroid and Head and Neck Surgery*,
https://doi.org/10.1007/978-3-031-24613-5_3

This Atlas is predominantly concerned with head and neck surgeries, and most of the neurophysiologic monitoring techniques required in these types of surgeries are designed to protect local peripheral cranial nerves and their branches that may be found during the course of these surgeries. The IONM techniques for monitoring of these peripheral cranial nerves and their branches predominantly consist of continuous free running EMG and stimulus triggered EMG.

Every muscle in the body is enervated by a nerve. When voluntarily or electrically stimulated, irritated or manipulated, the nerve sends a wave of electrical depolarization impulses along its length to the distal muscle it supplies. As this propagated nerve action potential reaches the motor end plate at the neuromuscular junction, the depolarizations are translated into motor unit action potentials (MUAPs) emanating from the corresponding muscle fibers. Summation of individual MUAPs results in a compound muscle action potential (CMAP) [1], which can then be electrically recorded by EMG. Modern IONM equipment will allow for both visualization and acoustical representation of these signals.

At rest, the nerve and muscle are electrically silent. With irritation or mechanical manipulation of a nerve, electrical discharges will be elicited by the nerve and can be recorded by electrodes placed at the corresponding muscle that the nerve enervates. These electrical discharges can consist of individual spike activity, bursts of spike activity, a train of regular repeating electrical activity, or neurotonic discharges representing a longer and more continuous set of rapid high frequency regular or irregular electrical discharges [2–4]. For free running continuous EMG, a nerve at rest and without stimulation or irritation should be electrically silent and not elicit any electrical activity. With traction, pressure, compression, or irritation of a nerve, the above neurotonic discharges can be detected with IONM with both visualization and acoustical representations of the above various electrical activities. When detected, this information can then be immediately relayed to the surgeon, whereby appropriate changes to the surgical procedure can then be undertaken to avoid further or permanent nerve related injury [5].

Triggered EMG allows the surgeon to individually stimulate neural and non-neural structures at various stimulus intensities throughout the surgical procedure, in order to document and map out whether a structure being stimulated is truly nerve related, and how this structure should be or should not be manipulated during the course of surgery. With electrical stimulation of a nerve via a sterile handheld probe by the surgeon, the muscle it innervates will produce an action potential which can then be electrically recorded. If an action potential is elicited after stimulation of the nerve, the surgeon is then informed that a response has been generated and stored, and that the structure being stimulated is indeed the nerve being monitored, which can then be mapped or avoided during the remainder of the course of surgery. If no action potential is elicited with triggered stimulation, then the structure being stimulated is most likely not the nerve being monitored. Unfortunately, false negatives can occur during direct stimulation of a nerve based on excessive anesthetic neuromuscular blockade, nerve hypothermia that can occur with cold water irrigation, altered and previously injured nerves being stimulated, neurophysiologic technical difficulties (electrode misplacement, faulty stimulation, recording equipment malfunction) [6], or proximal stimulation of a sharply transected nerve [7]. False positives may also occur with high stimulation intensities and current spread, metal objects crossing in the surgical field [8], light anesthesia, distal stimulation of a sharply transected nerve [7], other surgical instrumentation electrical artifact (i.e. electrocautery), 60 Hz electrical artifact, or preoperatively denervated muscle being used for recording [9].

In further chapters in this Atlas, various perspectives from specific members of the IONM team and specific monitoring procedures will be discussed, along with a following of pictorial examples of recorded responses from individual selected nerve monitoring cases.

## References


1. Kirchner ML, Kartush JM. Pitfalls in intraoperative nerve monitoring during vestibular schwannoma surgery. Neurosurg Focus. 2012;33:1–8.
2. Daube JS, Rubin DI. Needle electromyography. Muscle Nerve. 2009;39:24–270.
3. Lopez JR. Oculomotor and lower cranial nerve monitoring. In: Nuwer MR, editor. Intraoperative monitoring of neural function handbook of clinical neurophysiology, vol. 8; 2008. p. 385–95.
4. Crum BA, Strommen JA. Peripheral nerve stimulation and monitoring during operative procedures. Muscle Nerve. 2007;35:159–70.
5. Strommen JA, Crum BA. Intraoperative monitoring with free-running EMG. In: Nuwer MR, editor. Monitoring of neural function handbook of clinical neurophysiology, vol. 8; 2008. p. 396–403.
6. Holland NR. Intraoperative electromyography. J Clin Neurophysiol. 2004;19(5):444–53.
7. Nelson KR, Vasconez HC. Nerve transection without neurotonic discharges during intraoperative electromyographic monitoring. Muscle Nerve. 1995;18:236–8.
8. Pearlman RC, Isley MR, Ganey JC. Electrical artifact during intraoperative electromyographic neuromonitoring. Am J Electroneurodiagnostic Technol. 2008;48(2):107–18.
9. Coumans JVCE, Simon MV, Cooper JS, Winograd JM. Peripheral nerve surgery. In: Simon MV, editor. Intraoperative neurophysiology a comprehensive guide to monitoring and mapping; 2010. p. 267–98.

# Intraoperative Neurophysiological Monitoring Anesthesia Perspective

4

Hanna Kratochvil and Jeremy Goldfarb

## Introduction

General anesthetics aim to achieve the major goals of ensuring anxiolysis, amnesia, analgesia, unconsciousness, and autonomic areflexia. Thyroid and head and neck surgery requires an additional responsibility for anesthesia providers in the crucial partnership between the surgical team focused on intraoperative nerve monitoring (IONM). Laryngeal nerve monitoring endotracheal tubes have been advocated as a safety measure to prevent injury to laryngeal nerves. As the frequency of IONM increases, anesthesia technique is critical in improving quality and ultimately patient outcomes. This requires anesthesiologists to be familiar with specialized equipment setup, endotracheal tube placement, the monitoring system and parameters, as well as anesthetic technique.

## Preoperative Assessment

Preoperative examinations should include a general overview of the patient's comorbidities, functional status, and disease control. Evaluation for physical or functional obstruction including airway compression or deviation due to mass effect is crucial. Symptoms may include dysphagia, cough, or dyspnea that may worsen in the supine position. Imaging studies are also useful in this assessment and should routinely be reviewed. For patients with concerning risk factors, bedside nasal endoscopy or preoperative laryngeal examination (POLE) can be employed to visually assess the glottis (Fig. 4.1). This exam may help identify a deviated or narrowed airway, vocal cord injury, glottic edema, or significant dysphagia and is useful for perioperative planning and anticipating postoperative complications.

Inherited disorders of thyroid cancer must be considered in the setting of parathyroid, adrenal, or pituitary disease. Patients should be clinically euthyroid. Routine airway examination in addition to examination for possible tracheal deviation, stridor, or poor neck range of motion may identify a potentially difficult airway (Fig. 4.2).

Evaluation for underlying OSA is important in risk stratifying patients for potentially difficult masking on induction, employing opioid sparing techniques, and planning postoperative disposition. OSA symptoms may improve over time but are not likely to be observed immediately [1].

Anxiety levels may be high in anticipation of an upcoming procedure. In addition to impacting patient comfort, anxiety increases production of stress hormone, gastric secretions, and initial anesthetic requirements. Anxiolysis can be accomplished with benzodiazepines like midazolam and alpha 2 adrenergic agonists like dexmedetomidine or clonidine. If airway secretions are expected to be a concern, pretreatment with glycopyrrolate should be used. Employing a multimodal technique is warranted in these patients. Preoperative acetaminophen is appropriate for patients able to take oral medications. Dexmedetomidine may have opioid sparing properties and is a common adjunct to pain control. This has an added benefit of providing some element of neuroprotection in the aging patient [2].

H. Kratochvil (✉)
Massachusetts Eye and Ear, Harvard Medical School, Boston, MA, USA
e-mail: Hanna_Kratochvil@MEEI.Harvard.edu

J. Goldfarb
Massachusetts Eye and Ear, Inpatient Hospitalist Service, Harvard Medical School, Boston, MA, USA
e-mail: Jeremy_Goldfarb@MEEI.Harvard.edu


A. L. Shifrin et al. (eds.), *Atlas of Intraoperative Cranial Nerve Monitoring in Thyroid and Head and Neck Surgery*,
https://doi.org/10.1007/978-3-031-24613-5_4

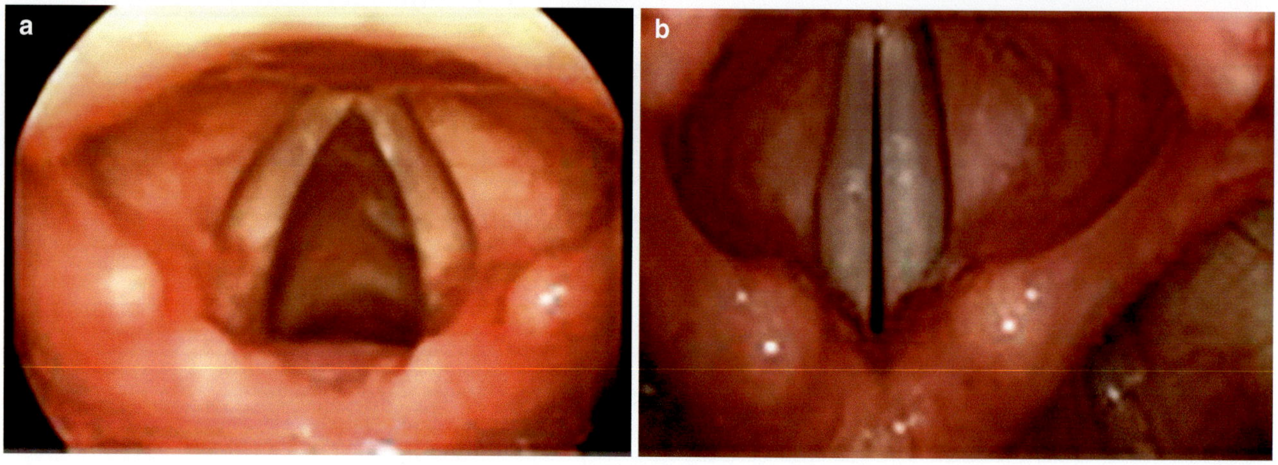


**Fig. 4.1** Preoperative laryngeal examination (POLE) revealing normal appearing glottis opening (**a**) and closing (**b**)

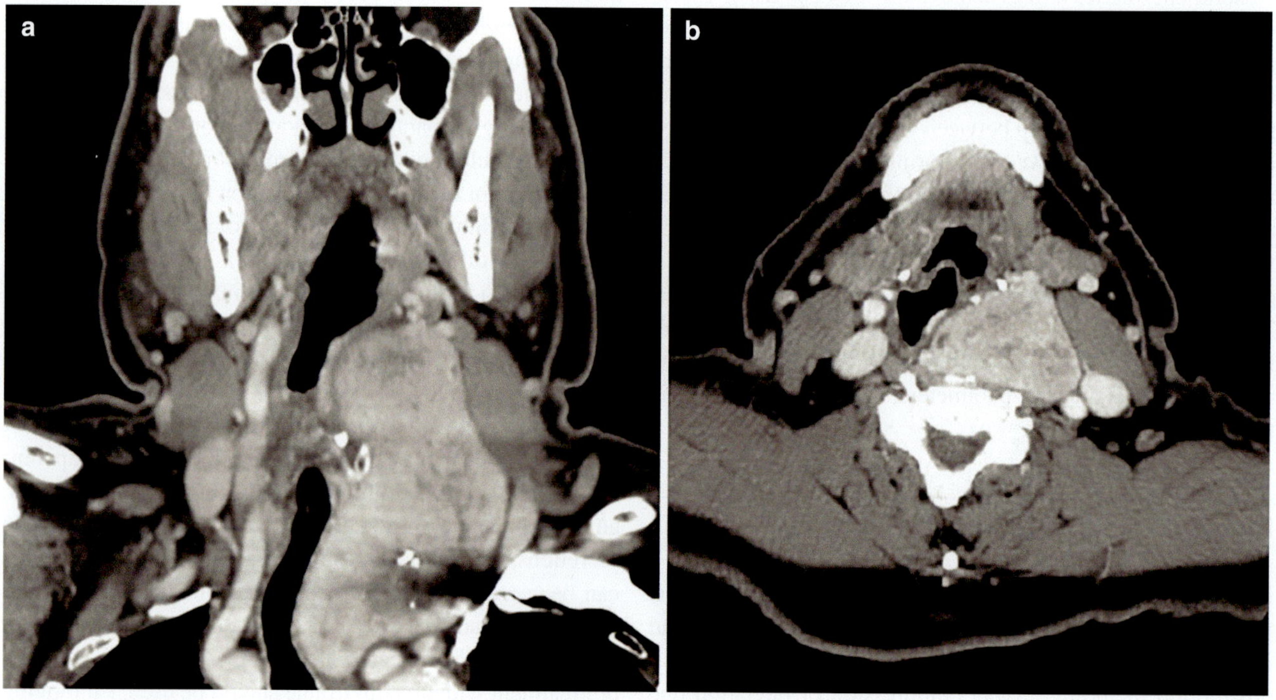


**Fig. 4.2** (**a**, **b**) CT scan images demonstrating large multinodular goiter causing significant deviation of the airway to the right. This anatomic deviation may raise additional concerns for securing the airway and should prompt further investigation

## Intraoperative Management

The appropriate placement of standard ASA monitors (additional monitoring as dictated by patient comorbidities), careful positioning, and preoxygenation should be performed. Many different induction techniques provide excellent intubation conditions with no deleterious effect on IONM. Combinations of propofol and a short acting opioid such as remifentanil 2–3 mcg/kg do not affect IONM. Short acting neuromuscular blockade with succinylcholine or rocuronium followed by reversal with sugammadex [3] can also be utilized to facilitate endotracheal intubation. Specialized nerve integrity monitoring (NIM) endotracheal tubes contain electrodes that are positioned at the vocal cords (Fig. 4.3). These electrodes transmit electromyographic signals to the receiver when the vocal cords contract. Both spontaneous and evoked electromyography (EMG) signals are recorded during thyroid surgery. The spontaneous EMG reports baseline recurrent laryngeal nerve activity. Evoked EMG is measured by direct stimulation of the vagus and recurrent laryngeal (RLN) nerves using low level pulsatile current, 1–2 milliamps. This current range has been established in both the pediatric and adult population [4, 5] (Fig. 4.4).

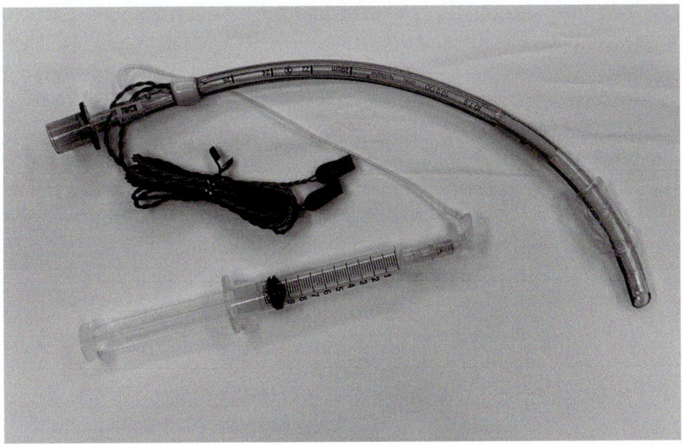

**Fig. 4.3** An example of a nerve integrity monitoring (NIM) endotracheal tube (ETT). Exposed electrodes line the sides of the area marked in blue. Some providers will include additional markings with an indelible pen to help establish the orientation of the tube after intubation and head positioning. This helps ensure bilateral symmetric contact with the vocal cords

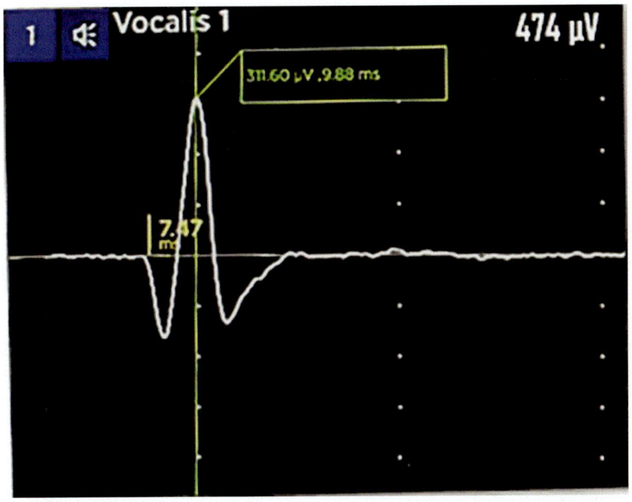


**Fig. 4.4** Stimulation of vagus nerve with appropriate electromyographic response

Additionally, repeated stimulation of both the Vagus and RLN intraoperatively has not been associated with nerve injury, fatigue, or hemodynamic consequences [6]. Video laryngoscopy is often employed to ensure proper placement of the NIM tube. This visualization is maintained during patient positioning as the tube may migrate proximally with head extension. Additional markings are sometimes drawn on the tube with an indelible marker to assist with alignment. Before initiating maintenance anesthesia, some providers will also allow the induction agents to metabolize (lightening the plane of anesthesia) until resumption of spontaneous RLN activity on the neural monitor can be seen. This provides another confirmatory sign of appropriate tube placement [7]. Both inhalation and total intravenous anesthesia (TIVA) techniques are appropriate for the maintenance of anesthesia, although the time to detection of a positive EMG signal during IONM appears to be shortened with TIVA technique [8].

Head and neck procedures require extension of the neck to achieve access to the surgical site. Caution must be taken during positioning as extreme extension can lead to nerve injury, vascular compromise, and even cardiac dysrhythmias from carotid body irritation [9, 10].

## Anesthesia Emergence

A smooth emergence is desirable in thyroid surgery patients as coughing or bucking may lead to hematoma formation and airway edema, which can develop both eccentrically and concentrically (the latter leading to potential airway compromise). An expanding hematoma should be immediately released by the surgical team with plans for an emergent re-intubation. Ensuring appropriate analgesia and utilizing remifentanil may facilitate a smooth emergence. Despite careful IONM, patients remain at risk for complications related to nerve injury. Unilateral nerve injuries usually produce voice changes but are not a threat to airway function. Bilateral recurrent laryngeal nerve injury can result in life threatening airway compromise as paralyzed vocal cords do not abduct during the respiratory cycle. This obstruction is only relieved by intubation or surgical airway.

## References

1. Schneider A, Bourahla K, Petiau C, Velten M, Volkmar PP, Rodier JF. Role of thyroid surgery in the obstructive sleep apnea syndrome. World J Surg. 2014;38(8):1990–4. https://doi.org/10.1007/s00268-014-2519-x. PMID: 24682279.
2. Ma D, Rajakumaraswamy N, Maze M. alpha2-adrenoceptor agonists: shedding light on neuroprotection? Br Med Bull. 2005;71:77–92. https://doi.org/10.1093/bmb/ldh036.
3. Donmez T, Erdem VM, Sunamak O, Ozcevik H. Thyroid surgery, IONM and sugammadex sodium relationships: benefits in sugammadex sodium use for Ionm. Acta Endocrinol (Buchar). 2019;15(4):454–9. https://doi.org/10.4183/aeb.2019.454. PMID: 32377242; PMCID: PMC7200106.
4. Chandrasekhar SS, Randolph GW, Seidman MD, Rosenfeld RM, Angelos P, Barkmeier-Kraemer J, et al. Clinical practice guideline: improving voice outcomes after thyroid surgery. Otolaryngol Head Neck Surg. 2013;148(6 Suppl):S1–S37.
5. Phelan E, Potenza A, Slough C, Zurakowski D, Kamani D, Randolph G. Recurrent laryngeal nerve monitoring during thyroid surgery: normative vagal and recurrent laryngeal nerve electrophysiological data. Otolaryngol Head Neck Surg. 2012;147(4):640–6.
6. White WM, Randolph GW, Hartnick CJ, Cunningham MJ. Recurrent laryngeal nerve monitoring during thyroidectomy and related cervical procedures in the pediatric population. Arch Otolaryngol Head Neck Surg. 2009;135(1):89–94.
7. Macias AA, Eappen S, Malikin I, Goldfarb J, Kujawa S, Konowitz PM, Kamani D, Randolph GW. Successful intraoperative electro-

physiologic monitoring of the recurrent laryngeal nerve, a multidisciplinary approach: The massachusetts eye and ear infirmary monitoring collaborative protocol with experience in over 3000 cases. Head Neck. 2016;38(10):1487–94. https://doi.org/10.1002/hed.24468. Epub 2016 Apr 9. PMID: 27062311.

8. Li X, Zhang B, Yu L, Yang J, Tan H. Influence of sevoflurane-based anesthesia versus total intravenous anesthesia on intraoperative neuromonitoring during thyroidectomy. Otolaryngol Head Neck Surg. 2020;162(6):853–9. https://doi.org/10.1177/0194599820912030. Epub 2020 Mar 17. PMID: 32178568.
9. Mercieri M, Paolini S, Mercieri A, De Blasi RA, Palmisani S, Pinto G, Arcioni R. Tetraplegia following parathyroidectomy in two long-term haemodialysis patients. Anesthesia. 2009;64:1010–3. (Lilitsis E, Papaioannou A, Hatzimichali A, et al. A case of asystole from carotid sinus hypersensitivity during patient positioning for thyroidectomy. BMC Anesthesiol. 2016;16(1):85). https://doi.org/10.1186/s12871-016-0255-5.
10. Suzuki T, Kurazumi T, Ueda T, Nagata H, Yamada T, Kosugi S, Hashiguchi S, Ito K, Morisaki H. Desflurane anesthesia worsens emergence agitation in adult patients undergoing thyroid surgery compared to sevoflurane anesthesia. JA Clin Rep. 2017;3(1):36. https://doi.org/10.1186/s40981-017-0106-5. Epub 2017 Jun 19. Retraction in: JA Clin Rep. 2020 Feb 14;6(1):13. PMID: 29457080; PMCID: PMC5804615.

# 5 Intraoperative Neurophysiological Monitoring Surgical Perspective

Christopher Blake Sullivan, Erivelto Volpi, and Joseph Scharpf

## Introduction

Thyroid surgery has been performed as early as 952 AD [1], and the volume of thyroid cancer and thyroid surgery continues to rapidly rise in recent decades [2, 3]. During thyroid surgery, the immediate locations of the recurrent laryngeal nerve (RLN) and external branch of the superior laryngeal nerve (EBSLN) put them at risk. Injury to the RLN is one of the most feared and significant complications during thyroid and parathyroid surgery and is one of the most common reasons for litigation after thyroid surgery [4]. Multiple studies have demonstrated that most RLN injuries occur due to traction at the ligament of Berry [5–7]. Other potential mechanisms of injury include compression, clamping, thermal, ligation, transection, and direct suctioning. The RLN serves multiple important factors due to motor and sensory fibers, and the motor fibers are responsible for adduction and abduction of the larynx. The EBSLN is composed of motor fibers that originate from the tenth cranial nerve and similarly provide motor innervation for the cricothyroid muscle and sensation for the supraglottis.

Intraoperative nerve monitoring (IONM) has been developed to help reduce risks to specific cranial nerves and was initially reported in the 1960s [8]. Modern IONM was introduced into thyroid surgery in the 1990s to help mitigate vocal cord palsy, and its application to the recurrent laryngeal nerve (RLN) is the most well-studied of the cranial nerves [9]. The gold standard for RLN monitoring is visual identification (Fig. 5.1) and IONM has become a common adjunct. As a result, the American Board of Otolaryngology-Head and Neck Surgery requires training in IONM for residents. The International Neural Monitoring Study Group (INMSG), a multidisciplinary group of surgeons and researchers, was founded in 2006 to help standardize guidance on the use of neurophysiologic monitoring during thyroid and parathyroid surgery. The American Academy of Otolaryngology-Head and Neck Surgery guidelines recommend IONM in cases of revision thyroid surgery, bilateral thyroid surgery, and in surgeries with only one functional RLN [10].

## Rationale for Intraoperative Nerve Monitoring

Routine thyroid and parathyroid surgery are safe operations with injury to the recurrent laryngeal nerve estimated to be 2% or less [4], but cranial nerve injury continues to be a

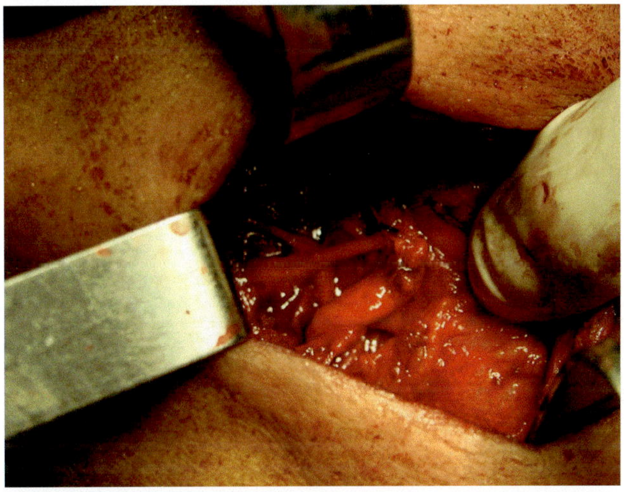

**Fig. 5.1** Right recurrent laryngeal nerve dissected, showing the inferior thyroid artery crossing the nerve posteriorly (*Courtesy of* Dr. Emerson Favero)

C. B. Sullivan
Department of Otolaryngology—Head and Neck Surgery, University of North Carolina, Chapel Hill, NC, USA

E. Volpi
Oncology Center of Hospital Alemao Oswaldo Cruz, Sao Paulo, Brazil

J. Scharpf (✉)
Head and Neck Institute, Cleveland Clinic Foundation, Cleveland, OH, USA
e-mail: scharpj@ccf.org


A. L. Shifrin et al. (eds.), *Atlas of Intraoperative Cranial Nerve Monitoring in Thyroid and Head and Neck Surgery*, https://doi.org/10.1007/978-3-031-24613-5_5

feared complication. Some studies show that RLN injury may be vastly underestimated due to heterogeneity in the utilization of pre- and post-operative laryngoscopy examination [9, 11]. Injury to the EBSLN has been reported to be as high as 58% [12], which often occurs when the superior thyroid pole and vessels are dissected. EBSLN injuries can lead to significant quality of life disturbances due to alteration in pitch. Unilateral vocal cord paralysis can lead to dysphonia, dysphagia, aspiration pneumonia, among many other adverse effects.

With IONM, the nerve of interest can be interrogated before, during, and after dissection. Previous studies have demonstrated nerve identification to be successful in 98% or greater in thyroid surgery when utilizing IONM [13]. Complication rates are similar when IONM is used by inexperienced surgeons compared to when an experienced surgeon assists [14]. After identification, intermittent use of IONM may help to reduce neuropraxia when meticulously dissecting out the RLN and associated branches (Fig. 5.2).

Multiple studies have also looked at prediction of post-operative vocal fold palsy during thyroid surgery with IONM [15]. Given the risk of RLN palsy is low, the positive predictive value for intermittent IONM is 37.8–80.5% and 47.6–88.2% for continuous IONM [15]. The negative predictive value is 97.3–99.8% for intermittent and 99.8–100% [15]. In an analysis of 3426 RLN at risk during thyroid surgery for benign disease, the sensitivity for detecting vocal cord dysfunction was 85.4% and the specificity was 99.0% [16]. Risk factors were not identified for false negative IONM procedures [16]. The true impact of IONM on preventing RLN paralysis is difficult to determine due to the lack of standardized guidelines, variability with pre- and post-operative laryngoscopy, and potential for inaccurate intraoperative amplitude response due to endotracheal tube migration.

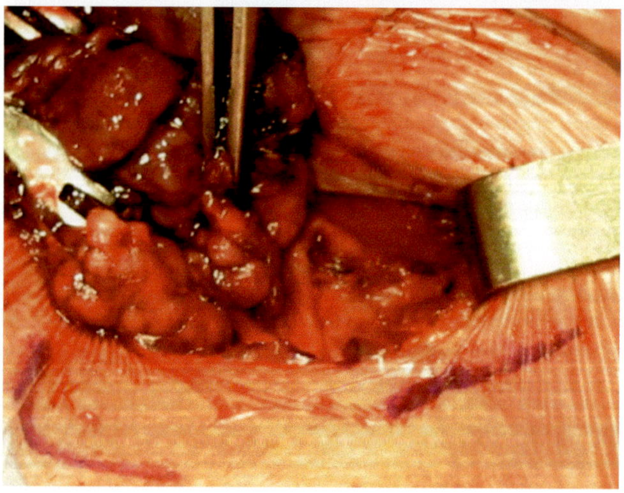

**Fig. 5.2** Traction of the recurrent laryngeal nerve due to its adherence to the thyroid gland. Traction is one of the most common causes of neuropraxia during thyroidectomy. IONM can prevent more severe nerve injuries and even change the surgical strategy

## Preventing Vocal Fold Injury

Improved or stable EMG signals during thyroid surgery suggest maintenance of the functional integrity of the RLN. Loss of IONM signal during total thyroidectomy cases can help provide valuable clinical information. According to the 2011 International Standards Guidelines Statement, a loss of satisfactory EMG signal is decrement of EMG activity with 100 μV or less, and no laryngeal twitch [13]. Steps need to be taken to assess whether a neural injury has occurred and if so to attempt to map the location of the injury. The surgeon will then need to decide whether or not to proceed to removal of the contralateral thyroid lobe [13]. A major advantage of IONM is to help predict possible bilateral vocal cord paralysis. Injury to both RLN can lead to severe airway complications, including the need for tracheostomy, future laryngeal reconstructive surgeries, and even death in extreme cases. If an ipsilateral nerve's functional status has deteriorated with IONM, then staged surgery at a later date can be considered. One study showed that injury to the RLN was only recognized in 1 of 6 patients undergoing bilateral thyroid surgery [11]. Another group showed that when a negative IONM signal was detected on the first side, the surgical plan was changed and there was no bilateral RLN injury compared to a group of patients where bilateral RLN injury occurred in 17% of patients when IONM was not utilized [17]. Melin et al. showed that 17% of patients developed bilateral vocal cord paralysis if surgery was continued on the contralateral side after a negative IONM signal on the initial side [18]. This compares to zero injuries to the RLN in the group where either surgery was terminated or staged to a later date. IONM has also been shown to be cost-effective for patients undergoing bilateral thyroid surgery [19]. In a survey of surgical departments in Germany performing bilateral thyroid surgery, over 90% of respondents indicated they would change their surgical plan to prevent bilateral vocal cord paralysis [20]. Only in very rare circumstances should surgery proceed to the contralateral side if there is an LOS with IONM on the initial side during thyroid surgery.

While LOS often indicates a vocal cord paralysis after surgery, incomplete LOS does not clearly correlate to post-operative vocal cord function [21]. This could potentially reflect a transient LOS, and post-operative laryngoscopy would not show any deficits. In certain cases, the LOS may be a false positive, which has been reported to be as high as 85% [22]. The false position of the EMG amplitude signal may be due to a variety of factors, including traction, movement of the endotracheal tube sense lead, and other variables which need to be considered.

Recurrent laryngeal nerve tumor infiltration is often seen with locally aggressive thyroid malignancies and can occur in up to 15% of patients with differentiated thyroid cancer [23]. Nerves that are involved by tumor require careful dissection due to their intimate involvement with tumor.

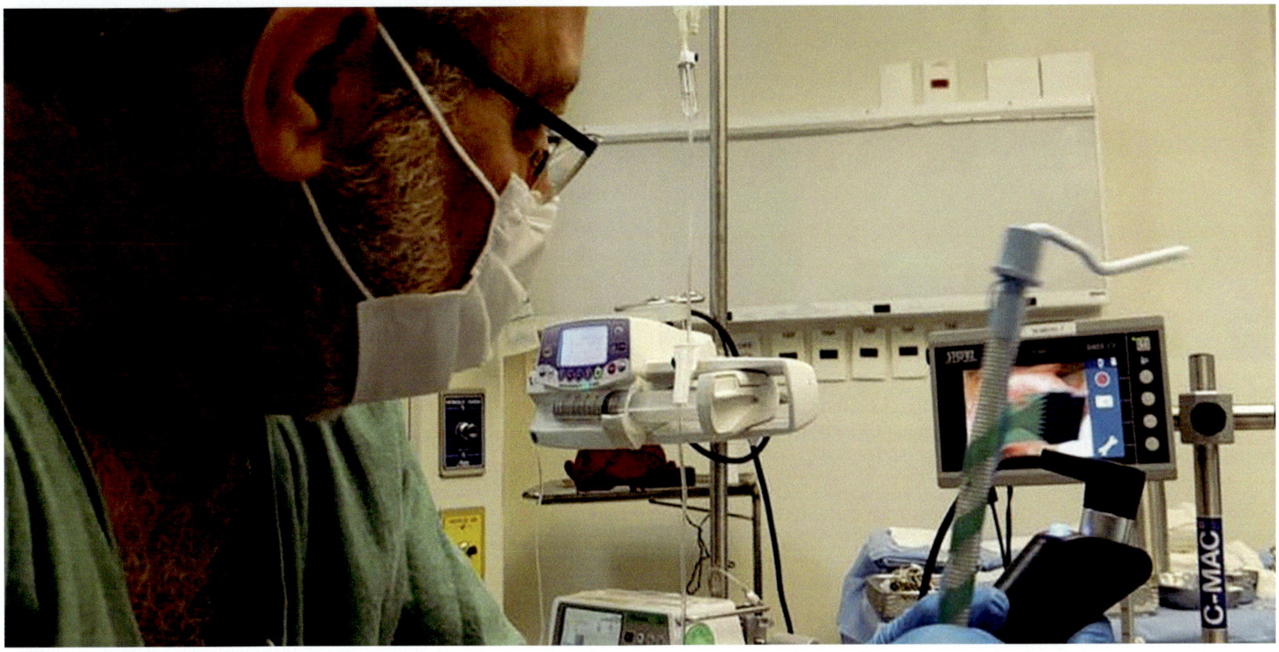


**Fig. 5.3** Example of an endotracheal tube-based recording system with surface electrodes; in this example, the electrodes are attached to the endotracheal tube

Intraoperative nerve monitoring is especially important in this subset of advanced cases due to the additional risk factors that may lead to RLN injury.

## Types of Intraoperative Nerve Monitoring

A variety of IONM systems have previously been used, and the most commonly employed system currently utilizes an endotracheal tube-based recording system with surface electrodes (Fig. 5.3). The goal of IONM is to stimulate a nerve of interest to produce muscle contraction and detectable electromyographic (EMG) waveform. The INMSG has previously published recommendations to standardize electrode recording systems for thyroid and parathyroid surgery [13]. Intermittent neural stimulation has been the mainstay for IONM, with continuous neural stimulation being less common. CIONM allows for real-time monitoring of the RLN when a probe is placed proximal to branching of the RLN on the vagus nerve. This provides the surgeon with an alert or change in the EMG waveform if an injury to the nerve occurs. Intermittent IONM produces an EMG waveform or muscle twitch when the nerve of interest or surrounding tissue is stimulated, and injury to the nerve usually occurs when the nerve is not being stimulated. In an analysis of 1526 patients who underwent thyroid surgery for benign disease, 788 patients had surgery using continuous IONM with no permanent vocal fold palsies compared to 4 of 738 patients ($p$ = 0.019) who had surgery with intermittent IONM. Both modalities of IONM provide the surgeon with helpful prognostic information of the RLN or EBSLN, which may help to facilitate next best treatment steps. Anterior laryngeal electrode systems have also been developed that obviate the need for an endotracheal based neural monitoring system [24].

## Safety of Intraoperative Nerve Monitoring

Intraoperative nerve monitoring has been shown to be safely applied without significant adverse events in thyroid and parathyroid surgery. Approximately 80% of head and neck surgeons utilize IONM during thyroid surgery [25]. Stimulation at 1–2 mA during intermittent or continuous IONM is similar to depolarization potentials with speaking [5]. An analysis of patients undergoing either continuous IONM or intermittent IONM showed greater vagal activity but this did not affect hemodynamics or increased release of the pro-inflammatory cytokine TNF-alpha [26]. For continuous IONM, safe surgery requires careful dissection, sometimes circumferentially, to place an electrode. While there have been few reports of adverse events with IONM [27], continuous or intermittent IONM has been shown to be overwhelmingly safe when used during thyroid or parathyroid surgery.

## Limitations

As with any technology, IONM is not without inherent limitations. Laryngeal based IONM with an endotracheal tube requires anesthesiologists who are familiar with the protocol necessary for nerve monitoring and proper placement of the

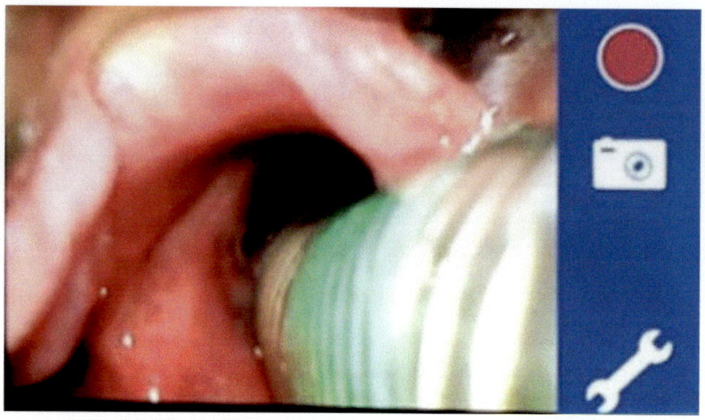

**Fig. 5.4** One of the strategies to correctly place the surface electrodes in contact with vocal folds is using a camera during the intubation. Here the anesthesiologist is using a camera in the laryngoscope for the best placement of the electrodes

endotracheal tube (Fig. 5.4). To date, there have been multiple studies that have questioned the value of IONM in helping to reduce RLN injuries [28, 29]. These variable results may be subject to a lack of statistical power. With intermittent IONM, the time between stimulations with a probe is not supervised, and the location and time of a neural injury may not be identified. CIONM aims to ameliorate this concern, but the results of CIONM vs intermittent IONM are not well-understood [30]. Movement of the endotracheal tube with the sense electrode can lead to a false positive LOS. During surgeries with IONM, signal loss has occurred an estimated 3.8–23% of the time [24].

## Conclusions

Injury to the RLN and EBSLN remains a significant concern during thyroid and parathyroid surgery. While visualization and anatomical knowledge of the RLN are the gold standard for functional preservation of the nerve, IONM is a safe adjunct and may be helpful in certain cases. IONM has the ability to help locate a neural injury during surgery and also to predict post-operative vocal cord function in select cases.

## References

1. Sarkar S, Banerjee S, Sarkar R, Sikder B. A review on the history of 'thyroid surgery'. Indian J Surg. 2016;78(1):32–6. https://doi.org/10.1007/s12262-015-1317-5.
2. Olson E, Wintheiser G, Wolfe KM, Droessler J, Silberstein PT. Epidemiology of thyroid cancer: a review of the national cancer database, 2000-2013. Cureus. 2019;11(2):e4127. https://doi.org/10.7759/cureus.4127.
3. Vaccarella S, Franceschi S, Bray F, Wild CP, Plummer M, Dal Maso L. Worldwide thyroid-cancer epidemic? The increasing impact of overdiagnosis. N Engl J Med. 2016;375(7):614–7. https://doi.org/10.1056/NEJMp1604412.
4. Abadin SS, Kaplan EL, Angelos P. Malpractice litigation after thyroid surgery: the role of recurrent laryngeal nerve injuries, 1989-2009. Surgery. 2010;148(4):718–22; discussion 722–3. https://doi.org/10.1016/j.surg.2010.07.019.
5. Schneider R, Randolph GW, Dionigi G, et al. International neural monitoring study group guideline 2018 part I: staging bilateral thyroid surgery with monitoring loss of signal. Laryngoscope. 2018;128:S1–S17. https://doi.org/10.1002/lary.27359.
6. Chiang F-Y, Lu I-C, Kuo W-R, Lee K-W, Chang N-C, Wu C-W. The mechanism of recurrent laryngeal nerve injury during thyroid surgery--the application of intraoperative neuromonitoring. Surgery. 2008;143(6):743–9. https://doi.org/10.1016/j.surg.2008.02.006.
7. Staubitz JI, Watzka F, Poplawski A, et al. Effect of intraoperative nerve monitoring on postoperative vocal cord palsy rates after thyroidectomy: European multicentre registry-based study. BJS Open. 2020;4(5):821–9. https://doi.org/10.1002/bjs5.50310.
8. Flisberg K, Lindholm T. Electrical stimulation of the human recurrent laryngeal nerve during thyroid operation. Acta Otolaryngol Suppl. 1969;263:63–7. https://doi.org/10.3109/00016487009131523.
9. Scharpf J, Liu JC, Sinclair C, et al. Critical review and consensus statement for neural monitoring in otolaryngologic head, neck, and endocrine surgery. Otolaryngol Head Neck Surg. 2021;166(2):233–48. https://doi.org/10.1177/01945998211011062.
10. Chandrasekhar SS, Randolph GW, Seidman MD, et al. Clinical practice guideline: improving voice outcomes after thyroid surgery. Otolaryngol Head Neck Surg. 2013;148(6 Suppl):S1–37. https://doi.org/10.1177/0194599813487301.
11. Bergenfelz A, Jansson S, Kristoffersson A, et al. Complications to thyroid surgery: results as reported in a database from a multicenter audit comprising 3,660 patients. Langenbeck's Arch Surg. 2008;393(5):667–73. https://doi.org/10.1007/s00423-008-0366-7.
12. Jansson S, Tisell LE, Hagne I, Sanner E, Stenborg R, Svensson P. Partial superior laryngeal nerve (SLN) lesions before and after thyroid surgery. World J Surg. 1988;12(4):522–7. https://doi.org/10.1007/BF01655439.
13. Randolph GW, Dralle H, International Intraoperative Monitoring Study Group, et al. Electrophysiologic recurrent laryngeal nerve monitoring during thyroid and parathyroid surgery: international standards guideline statement. Laryngoscope. 2011;121(Suppl):S1–16. https://doi.org/10.1002/lary.21119.
14. Alesina PF, Hinrichs J, Meier B, Cho EY, Bolli M, Walz MK. Intraoperative neuromonitoring for surgical training in thyroid surgery: its routine use allows a safe operation instead of lack of experienced mentoring. World J Surg. 2014;38(3):592–8. https://doi.org/10.1007/s00268-013-2372-3.
15. Schneider R, Machens A, Lorenz K, Dralle H. Intraoperative nerve monitoring in thyroid surgery-shifting current paradigms. Gland Surg. 2020;9(Suppl 2):S120–8. https://doi.org/10.21037/gs.2019.11.04.
16. Melin M, Schwarz K, Pearson MD, Lammers BJ, Goretzki PE. Postoperative vocal cord dysfunction despite normal intraoperative neuromonitoring: an unexpected complication with the risk of bilateral palsy. World J Surg. 2014;38(10):2597–602. https://doi.org/10.1007/s00268-014-2591-2.
17. Goretzki PE, Schwarz K, Brinkmann J, Wirowski D, Lammers BJ. The impact of intraoperative neuromonitoring (IONM) on surgical strategy in bilateral thyroid diseases: is it worth the effort? World J Surg. 2010;34(6):1274–84. https://doi.org/10.1007/s00268-009-0353-3.
18. Melin M, Schwarz K, Lammers BJ, Goretzki PE. IONM-guided goiter surgery leading to two-stage thyroidectomy--indication and results. Langenbeck's Arch Surg. 2013;398(3):411–8. https://doi.org/10.1007/s00423-012-1032-7.
19. Al-Qurayshi Z, Kandil E, Randolph GW. Cost-effectiveness of intraoperative nerve monitoring in avoidance of bilateral recurrent laryngeal nerve injury in patients undergoing total thyroidec-

tomy. Br J Surg. 2017;104(11):1523–31. https://doi.org/10.1002/bjs.10582.

20. Dralle H, Sekulla C, Lorenz K, Nguyen Thanh P, Schneider R, Machens A. Loss of the nerve monitoring signal during bilateral thyroid surgery. Br J Surg. 2012;99(8):1089–95. https://doi.org/10.1002/bjs.8831.
21. Yuan Q, Wu G, Hou J, Liao X, Liao Y, Chiang F-Y. Correlation between electrophysiological changes and outcomes of vocal cord function in 1764 recurrent laryngeal nerves with visual integrity during thyroidectomy. Thyroid. 2020;30(5):739–45. https://doi.org/10.1089/thy.2019.0361.
22. Sitges-Serra A, Fontané J, Dueñas JP, et al. Prospective study on loss of signal on the first side during neuromonitoring of the recurrent laryngeal nerve in total thyroidectomy. Br J Surg. 2013;100(5):662–6. https://doi.org/10.1002/bjs.9044.
23. Wu C-W, Dionigi G, Barczynski M, et al. International neuromonitoring study group guidelines 2018: part II: optimal recurrent laryngeal nerve management for invasive thyroid cancer-incorporation of surgical, laryngeal, and neural electrophysiologic data. Laryngoscope. 2018;128(Suppl):S18–27. https://doi.org/10.1002/lary.27360.
24. Liddy W, Lawson BR, Barber SR, et al. Anterior laryngeal electrodes for recurrent laryngeal nerve monitoring during thyroid and parathyroid surgery: new expanded options for neural monitoring. Laryngoscope. 2018;128(12):2910–5. https://doi.org/10.1002/lary.27362.
25. Al-Qurayshi Z, Randolph GW, Alshehri M, Kandil E. Analysis of variations in the use of intraoperative nerve monitoring in thyroid surgery. JAMA Otolaryngol Neck Surg. 2016;142(6):584. https://doi.org/10.1001/jamaoto.2016.0412.
26. Friedrich C, Ulmer C, Rieber F, et al. Safety analysis of vagal nerve stimulation for continuous nerve monitoring during thyroid surgery. Laryngoscope. 2012;122(9):1979–87. https://doi.org/10.1002/lary.23411.
27. Terris DJ, Chaung K, Duke WS. Continuous vagal nerve monitoring is dangerous and should not routinely be done during thyroid surgery. World J Surg. 2015;39(10):2471–6. https://doi.org/10.1007/s00268-015-3139-9.
28. Cirocchi R, Arezzo A, D'Andrea V, et al. Intraoperative neuromonitoring versus visual nerve identification for prevention of recurrent laryngeal nerve injury in adults undergoing thyroid surgery. Cochrane Database Syst Rev. 2019;1:CD012483. https://doi.org/10.1002/14651858.CD012483.pub2.
29. Zheng S, Xu Z, Wei Y, Zeng M, He J. Effect of intraoperative neuromonitoring on recurrent laryngeal nerve palsy rates after thyroid surgery--a meta-analysis. J Formos Med Assoc. 2013;112(8):463–72. https://doi.org/10.1016/j.jfma.2012.03.003.
30. Choi SY, Son Y-I. Intraoperative neuromonitoring for thyroid surgery: the proven benefits and limitations. Clin Exp Otorhinolaryngol. 2019;12(4):335–6. https://doi.org/10.21053/ceo.2019.00542.

# Electrophysiologic RLN and Vagal Monitoring During Thyroid and Parathyroid Surgery

6

Amanda Silver Karcioglu, Marika D. Russell, Amr H. Abdelhamid Ahmed, and Gregory W. Randolph

## Introduction

### Brief History of IONM

The recurrent laryngeal nerve (RLN) and external branch of the superior laryngeal nerve (EBSLN, discussed in a separate chapter) are at risk during thyroid and parathyroid surgery. Injury to the RLN can significantly impact quality of life, altering the ability to speak, swallow, and/or breathe. The importance of preservation of the RLN dates back to the second century when Galen identified these nerves as contributing to vocal production and termed them "reversivi" or recurrent nerves, noting their reversal of descent into the chest with ascent back into the neck [1].

Successful management and preservation of the RLN during thyroid and parathyroid surgery requires a thorough understanding of vagus nerve (VN) and RLN anatomy. Kocher and Billroth sought to avoid the nerve to prevent injury [2]. Thereafter, visual identification during surgical dissection, attributed to August Bier (Berlin) in 1911 [2], Frank Lahey (Boston) in 1938 [3], and later VH Riddell (London) in 1956 [4] became regarded as the gold standard for nerve preservation. However, there is strong evidence that visual identification alone is insufficient and does not ensure laryngeal function postoperatively [5–7].

Over time, various adjunctive methods have been used to augment visual identification with incorporation of functional assessment. In 1966, endotracheal tubes adapted to detect glottic movement via pressure changes in a balloon placed at the level of the glottis were described in canine RLN models [8]. In 1969, Flisberg and Lindholm described successful RLN intraoperative nerve monitoring in 13 patients (15 nerves) using needle electrodes inserted into the vocalis muscle through the cricothyroid membrane to record muscle action potentials. Nerve conduction velocities for each nerve were also calculated [9]. Contemporaneously, Riddell described RLN monitoring with electrical stimulation of the RLN, utilizing intraoperative direct laryngoscopy for glottic evaluation to confirm function prior to proceeding with the second side during total thyroidectomy [10]. In 1981, Engel et al. applied a double-cuff endotracheal tube to monitor pressure changes at the level of the glottis; however, high cuff pressures required at the trachea limited broader adoption [11]. Around the same time, in order to circumvent the need for complex instrumentation, Gavilan described direct palpation of the posterior cricoarytenoid muscle during nerve stimulation as a simplified method of RLN monitoring [12] and James described ipsilateral laryngeal palpation during RLN stimulation [13].

In 1988, the Nerve Integrity Monitoring system (NIM-2), a system that offered both visual and auditory feedback with background and evoked EMG, was introduced by the company Xomed-Treace. In 1991, Rice and Cone-Wesson were the first to describe using a Prass monopolar nerve stimulator probe with the NIMS-2 system for RLN monitoring [14]. Their method involved endoscopically placed hook wires in the vocalis muscle. In 1996, Eisele reported on the use of a novel simplified endotracheal tube with integrated stainless-steel-wire surface electrodes (NIM-2 EMG endotracheal tube) for RLN monitoring in lieu of intramus-

A. S. Karcioglu
Division of Otolaryngology—Head and Neck Surgery, Department of Surgery, NorthShore University HealthSystem, Evanston, IL, USA

The University of Chicago, Pritzker School of Medicine, Chicago, IL, USA

M. D. Russell · A. H. Abdelhamid Ahmed
Division of Thyroid and Parathyroid Endocrine Surgery, Department of Otolaryngology—Head and Neck Surgery, Massachusetts Eye and Ear Infirmary, Harvard Medical School, Boston, MA, USA
e-mail: Amr_Ahmed@meei.harvard.edu

G. W. Randolph (✉)
Otolaryngology Head and Neck Surgery, Claire and John Bertucci Endowed Chair in Thyroid Surgical Oncology, Harvard Medical School, Boston, MA, USA
e-mail: Gregory_Randolph@meei.harvard.edu



A. L. Shifrin et al. (eds.), *Atlas of Intraoperative Cranial Nerve Monitoring in Thyroid and Head and Neck Surgery*,
https://doi.org/10.1007/978-3-031-24613-5_6

cular electrodes [15]. With its commercial availability and user-friendly hardware, this reliable system, currently in its third generation (NIM-3 Response, Medtronic, Xomed, Jacksonville, FL) remains the most commonly used for RLN monitoring today.

## Prevalence and Patterns of IONM Use

Since its early description over 50 years ago [9, 10] intraoperative nerve monitoring (IOMN) has gained increased acceptance as an adjunctive technique for RLN preservation, offering a dynamic functional assessment of the RLN. Surveys conducted over a decade ago found adoption rates of 37–45% among both general surgeons and otolaryngologist head and neck surgeons [16, 17]. Over time, utilization has steadily increased. Marti et al. reported 95% of respondents used IONM (60% routinely and 35% selectively) in a survey of the American Association of Endocrine Surgeons (AAES) and the American Head and Neck Society (AHNS) [18]. A recent international survey of the American Academy of Otolaryngology-Head and Neck Surgery, International Association of Endocrine Surgeons, and AHNS found 83% of the 1015 respondents reported using IONM, with over 65% always using IONM, 18% using it in select cases, and up to 95% reporting use in reoperative cases [19]. In this study, usage varied by geographic location, with 70% of North American surgeons reporting use of IONM compared to 27% of non-North American surgeons. German surveys have noted higher rates of utilization, with IONM being employed in 91% of thyroidectomies across a survey of German surgical centers in 2012 [20]. In a more recent German multicenter survey of 12,888 patients (18,793 nerves at risk) receiving surgery for benign goiter, IONM was used 98% of cases [21].

Feng et al. demonstrated that younger surgeons and those with <15 years of practice were more likely to use IOMN, similar to findings in earlier studies [16, 17, 22]. This suggests exposure to the technology may increase usage and may also reflect a more general growing acceptance of IOMN [19]. High volume surgeons (>100 cases per year) and fellowship-trained endocrine and head and neck surgeons report higher rates of IONM [17, 18, 23], possibly reflecting an understanding of the inherent challenge of predicting preoperatively which cases might benefit most from IONM. Surgeons reporting always using IONM (in contrast to selected usage of IONM) were two times more likely to adjust surgical extent by not completing a total thyroidectomy if loss of signal (LOS) was noted [18], suggesting increased familiarity with the technology facilitates application by improving interpretation and ability to troubleshoot when needed [24].

## Role in Education

Utilization of IONM enables the surgeon to interrogate nerve anatomy and function with immediate quantitative feedback, thereby augmenting surgical training. Importantly, surgical skills and sound anatomic knowledge remain prerequisite and are not supplanted by IONM use. Application of IONM in head and neck surgery, including indications, techniques, and pitfalls, is required for residents in otolaryngology-head and neck surgery programs [25]. For those receiving fellowship training under the supervision of the AHNS or the AAES, thorough understanding and ability to perform IONM of the RLN is required [26, 27]. As exposure to IONM during training has been shown to be associated with higher utilization by surgeons upon entering practice independently [17, 18], continued increase in utilization is expected. Nonetheless, there remains inconsistency globally in training and application. The International Neuromonitoring Study Group (INMSG) has been at the forefront of IONM technology and adoption and recently published a consensus statement addressing the recommended essential components of training courses to support optimal implementation and practice [28].

## Rationale and Indications for IONM

### Rates and Impact of Vocal Cord Paralysis

Rates of RLN injury during thyroid and parathyroid surgery are imprecise and likely underreported due to the lack of systematic and standardized pre- and postoperative direct laryngeal evaluation. Lack of standardization with respect to surgical complexity and surgeon experience further complicates understanding. Historically, rates of RLN injury have been reported to be quite low, with temporary RLN injury reported to occur in 5–8% of cases and permanent RLN paralysis reported to occur in 0.3–3% of cases [29]. In a systematic review of 25,000 patients, temporary RLN injury occurred in 9.8% and permanent RLN paralysis occurred in 2.3% of cases, though depending on the method of laryngeal evaluation, overall postoperative vocal cord paralysis (VCP) ranged from 2.3% to 26% [30]. With routine postoperative laryngeal examination, detected rates of postoperative VCP were found to double in analysis of two large national databases (Scandinavian Quality Register and British Association of Endocrine and Thyroid Surgeons Audit) [31, 32].

Fortunately, bilateral VCP is rare, reported to occur in 0.1–1.3% of thyroid surgery [33–35]. In a study of over 7000 patients, Sarkis et al. reported a bilateral VCP rate of 0.1% and concluded IOMN can be a useful adjunct during surgery, allowing for staged surgery when LOS occurs [33] as endorsed by the INMSG [7].

Injury to the RLN may present with a range of clinical complaints. Neural dysfunction resulting from injury to small branches of the RLN may not be associated with a visible vocal fold abnormality but may manifest as cough, globus, or dysphagia [36]. When frank VCP occurs, it may present with dysphonia, aspiration, dysphagia, and dyspnea, symptoms which may alter quality of life and impair one's ability to work [37, 38]. Moreover, VCP may be associated with significant emotional or psychological distress, with patients experiencing frustration, isolation, fear, and an altered sense of identity [36].

## Role of Preoperative Laryngeal Examination

Routine preoperative laryngeal examination is not universally performed but is increasingly recognized as an essential component of thyroid and parathyroid surgical care. The sensitivity of voice change to screen for VCP ranges from 33% to 68% [39–41], underscoring the importance of direct pre- and postoperative laryngeal examination. Several professional organizations have published recommendations for standardizing practice of laryngeal examination. The AHNS, American Academy of Otolaryngology-Head and Neck Surgery (AAO-HNS) and American Thyroid Association (ATA) have all recommended preoperative laryngeal examination for patients undergoing thyroid surgery who are at risk of RLN injury or involvement by tumor, including those with preoperative voice abnormality, a history of prior surgery placing the RLN or vagus nerve at risk, or malignancy with posterior extrathyroidal extension or bulky central neck adenopathy [42–44]. The AHNS recommends preoperative laryngeal examination for all patients with thyroid malignancy [43, 45] and the German Association of Endocrine Surgeons recommends preoperative and postoperative laryngoscopy for all patients receiving thyroid surgery [46]. The INMSG acknowledges that knowledge of preoperative laryngeal function is essential for optimal use of IONM and recommends preoperative and postoperative laryngoscopy for all patients receiving neuromonitored thyroid surgery [47].

## Evidence Basis for Benefit of IONM

Assessing the impact of IOMN on rates of RLN injury in thyroid and parathyroid surgery is hindered by several factors, including variability of preoperative and postoperative laryngeal evaluation and lack of standardization across studies evaluating rates of nerve injury with and without IOMN. To address this variability and promote standards of IONM use, INMSG developed an International Standard Guidelines Statement in 2011 [47]. Lack of high-level evidence demonstrating a benefit also stems in part from the low incidence of reported or identified RLN injury. Assessing the statistical power needed to prove lower rates of RLN paralysis using IONM, and using generally accepted reported rates of paralysis, Dralle calculated a requirement of 9,000,000 patients per arm for benign multinodular goiter, and approximately 40,000 patients per arm for thyroid cancer [2].

Meta-analyses examining the impact of IONM on rates of VCP have yielded conflicting results. Zheng et al. demonstrated decreased transient rates of VCP with use of IONM, whereas meta-analyses performed by Higgins et al. and Pisanu et al. found no impact of IONM VCP rates [48–50]. In a systematic review and meta-analysis evaluating over 17,200 nerves at risk, Yang et al. found benefit (without statistical significance) in using IOMN to reduce the incidence of RLN injury and reduce the amount of residual thyroid tissue in patients undergoing total thyroidectomy for thyroid cancer [51]. A recent study analyzing 4598 cases of thyroidectomy from a European registry identified a lower risk of postoperative VCP when IONM was used (0.9% with IONM versus 3.1% without IONM) [52].

The benefit of IONM in high-risk surgical groups may be more readily demonstrated. A meta-analysis performed by Wong et al. found decreased rates of transient RLN paralysis in surgeries for malignancy and decreased rates of overall RLN paralysis in reoperative cases [53]. In a retrospective study of 850 patients who underwent reoperative thyroid and parathyroid surgery, Barczyski et al. found decreased rates of transient RLN paralysis with use of IONM [54]. A randomized study of 1000 patients found a statistically significant lower rate of transient RLN paralysis in cases judged to be at high-risk of RLN injury, including those with anatomic branching patterns [55].

Despite the relative lack of high-level evidence demonstrating improved outcomes with IONM, neural monitoring is endorsed by several international societies. The INMSG recommends using IOMN in thyroid surgery to help identify, map, and preserve the RLN well as guide intraoperative management of the invaded RLN [47, 56]. The AHNS has published a consensus statement for management of RLN during thyroidectomy which recommends preoperative direct laryngeal evaluation and use of IONM [57]. The German Association of Endocrine Surgery Guidelines similarly endorse the use of IOMN as an adjunct to the gold standard of visual identification [46].

## IONM Standards of Use and Applications

To promote uniform and optimal application of IONM, the INMSG published a comprehensive two-part set of guidelines in 2018 outlining standards of use (Table 6.1) [7, 56]. The major applications and benefits of IONM are summarized as follows:

**Table 6.1** The international RLN anatomic classification and estimated prevalence of each class

| Class | Description | Prevalence |
|---|---|---|
| *I/II: Left/right RLN basic surgical anatomic path* | | |
| L1/R1 | Normal trajectory | 95/90% |
| L2a/R2a | Abnormal acquired—lateral/medial | 5/5–10% |
| L2b/R2b | Abnormal acquired—ventral | <1%/<1% |
| L3/R3 | Abnormal embryologic—nonrecurrent | 0.04%/0.5–1% |
| *III: Clinically important neural features* | | |
| *Anatomical* | | |
| F—Fixed/splayed/entrapped | Capsular association through fascial bands, vessels, or goitrous change | 15% (with substernal goiter) |
| I—Invaded | Neural invasion | <5% (with cancer) |
| L—Posterior ligament | Posterior ligament of Berry or associated vessel neural entrapment | 10% |
| B—Branched | Extralaryngeal RLN branching | 24.3–72% |
| T—Thin | Neural caliber <1 mm | <2.5% |
| *Dynamic* | | |
| LOS—Loss of signal | Loss of EMG signal | |
| D—Extensive neural dissection | Extensive nerve dissection or 360° dissection | |

*RLN* recurrent laryngeal nerve, *EMG* electromyographic, *LOS* loss of signal

Reproduced with permission from *The Recurrent and Superior Laryngeal Nerves*, Chapter 12, Randolph GW, Ed, copyright Springer Nature

**Table 6.2** Key elements of neuromonitoring use during various phases of surgery

| | |
|---|---|
| Set-up | • Confirm correct placement of ETT with respiratory variation or videolaryngoscopy<br>• Place grounding electrodes, connect all electrodes to interface-connector box<br>• Check impedance values, set stimulating current to 1–2 mA, event threshold to 100 μV |
| Initiation of surgery | • Stimulate strap muscles to observe gross muscle twitch, confirm absence of neuromuscular blockade<br>• Identify carotid sheath, stimulate vagus nerve, and confirm baseline response of >500 μV and detectable laryngeal twitch |
| Surgery proceeds | • Electrical stimulation used for neural mapping, differentiating neural from nonneural tissue, confirming RLN<br>• Observe for adverse EMG changes; if amplitude decreases >50% and latency increases >10% from baseline, halt or modify surgical maneuver |
| Potential loss of signal | • Observe for presence of laryngeal twitch<br>• If laryngeal twitch is present, consider recording side error; adjust ETT, check electrode connections<br>• If laryngeal twitch is absent, consider stimulating side error; ensure a dry field, confirm absence of neuromuscular blockade, test contralateral vagus nerve |
| Loss of signal | • If LOS is confirmed to be present at termination of the first side, allow a 20-min waiting period for neural recovery<br>• If signal recovers to >50% of initial baseline and >250 μV, proceed with contralateral side<br>• If complete recovery criteria are not met, consider staging contralateral surgery |

*ETT* endotracheal tube, *RLN* recurrent laryngeal nerve, *EMG* electromyography, *LOS* loss of signal

1. Intraoperative mapping, dissection, and identification of the RLN

   The use of electrical neural mapping facilitates visual identification of the RLN. Prior to direct visualization, the approximate location and course of the nerve is mapped in the paratracheal region through electrical stimulation, facilitating focused dissection and subsequent visual identification. Differentiating neural vs nonneural structures through IONM permits identification of anatomic variants such as the anterior motor branch, which should be recognized in the setting of an extralaryngeal branching pattern [7]. IONM provides additional aid in mapping and identifying nerve in the setting of scar tissues and distorted anatomy frequently encountered in reoperative cases.
2. Intraoperative identification of impending neuropraxic injury and elucidation of mechanism of injury

   Evolving EMG changes observed during surgical manipulation can predict impending neuropraxia, allowing opportunity to cease injurious maneuvers and avoid severe neural injury [58, 59]. If neuropraxic injury occurs, retrograde stimulation along the course of the nerve can be used to identify the injured segment, illuminating the likely mechanism of injury and providing a learning opportunity for the surgeon.
3. Prognostication of neural function

   Following completion of the initial surgical side, electrical stimulation can be used to determine the functional status of the RLN. This allows the surgeon to determine whether contralateral surgery should be staged in order to avoid risk of bilateral VCP.
4. Management of the invaded RLN

   Intraoperative neuromonitoring data can be combined with surgical information and overall patient and disease characteristics to guide surgical management of the invaded RLN (Table 6.2).

## Surgical Anatomy of the Vagus/RLN

### Normal Anatomy

Knowledge of the anatomy and, importantly, variability in the position of the VN and RLN, is prerequisite to safe thyroid and parathyroid surgery and optimal use of IONM. In most patients, the common carotid artery (CCA) is located medially to the VN, with the internal jugular vein (IJV) anterolaterally or laterally positioned within the carotid sheath. Less commonly, the IJV can be found medially [60, 61]. In 2010, Dionigi et al. published an anatomical classification of the VN which provides a reproducible method for identifying the VN within the carotid sheath based on its position relative to the great vessels (CCA and IJV) [61]. In this classification, an anterior VN (with respect to the great vessels) is denoted by the letter **A** (4% of cases)**,** a posterior VN (with respect to the great vessels) is denoted by the letter **P** (73% of cases), a VN posterior to the IJV (8% of cases) is denoted by **Pj**, and a VN posterior to the CCA (8%) by **Pc**. This classification is useful for locating the VN during IONM.

The anatomical position of the right and left RLN differs due to early embryological development, wherein the RLN is pulled down by the lowest persistent aortic arch. On the right, the RLN courses from the posterior aspect of the carotid sheath in the neck base and loops from anterior to posterior around the first segment of the subclavian artery (the fourth branchial arch remnant) before crossing obliquely from lateral to medial as it ascends the neck to the larynx. On the left, however, the RLN branches underneath the aortic arch (sixth arch, ligamentum arteriosus) just lateral to the obliterated ductus arteriosus before ascending to the larynx in a direct cranial-caudal path within the tracheoesophageal (TE) groove. Thus, in over 80% of subjects, the right RLN follows in a more oblique path to the larynx (15–45° relative to the TE groove compared to the left RLN, which travels parallel to the TE groove at an angle <30°) (**R1 and L1**, see Fig. 6.1, Table 6.3).

## Variant Anatomy

Variations in RLN anatomy may be embryologic or acquired and place the RLN at risk during surgery. Randolph et al. have published a surgical anatomic classification of the RLN describing normal anatomy along with embryological and acquired variations [62], as depicted in Fig. 6.2 and Table 6.1. Goitrous enlargement may displace the RLN, producing acquired variation; the left RLN may be displaced laterally when the goiter extends into the TE groove (**L2a**); the right RLN may be displaced medially by goitrous enlargement of the dorsal or mid-inferior pole of the thyroid, causing it to course more parallel to the TE groove at an angle <15° (**R2a**). The RLN can also be displaced ventrally if thyroid tissue, particularly the tubercle of Zuckerkandl, enlarges deep to the trachea, as with retrotracheal or posterior mediastinal goiters (**L2b or Rb2**).

Careful study of cross-sectional imaging prior to surgery can alert the surgeon to the possibility of a nonrecurrent RLN, which occurs in less than 1% of patients but poses sig-

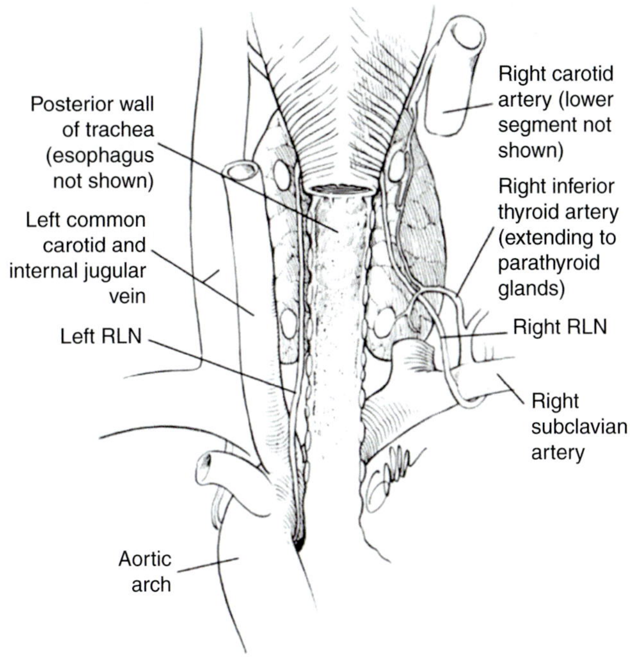


**Fig. 6.1** Posterior view of the right and left RLN. The right RLN traverses superiorly in a more oblique course than the left RLN which travels in the tracheoesophageal groove. *RLN* recurrent laryngeal nerve. (Reproduced with permission from *Surgery of the Thyroid and Parathyroid Glands, 3rd Ed.* Chapter 36; Fig. 36.3 A. Randolph, GW, Ed, copyright Elsevier)

**Table 6.3** Algorithms for management of the invaded recurrent laryngeal nerve based on preoperative laryngeal function

| Management of the invaded RLN | |
|---|---|
| Preoperative laryngeal examination | Recommended strategy |
| Intact vocal cord mobility | • Start with dominant side<br>• Superficial involvement: Shave resection where feasible<br>• Extensive involvement: Determine RLN preservation vs. resection based on disease- and patient-specific factors |
| Ipsilateral vocal cord paralysis | • Start with contralateral side<br>• If LOS on contralateral side, await possible intraoperative recovery<br>• If no LOS on contralateral side, use proximal stimulability of invaded RLN to determine appropriateness of preservation vs. resection<br>• If no proximal stimulability, resect RLN<br>• If proximal stimulability is intact, determine RLN preservation vs. resection based on disease- and patient-specific factors |
| Contralateral vocal cord paralysis | • Determine whether observation or non-surgical treatment is a feasible option<br>• If proceeding with surgery, perform careful shave resection with plan for adjuvant treatment<br>• Resect nerve and perform tracheotomy in rare cases |

*LOS* loss of signal, *RLN* recurrent laryngeal nerve

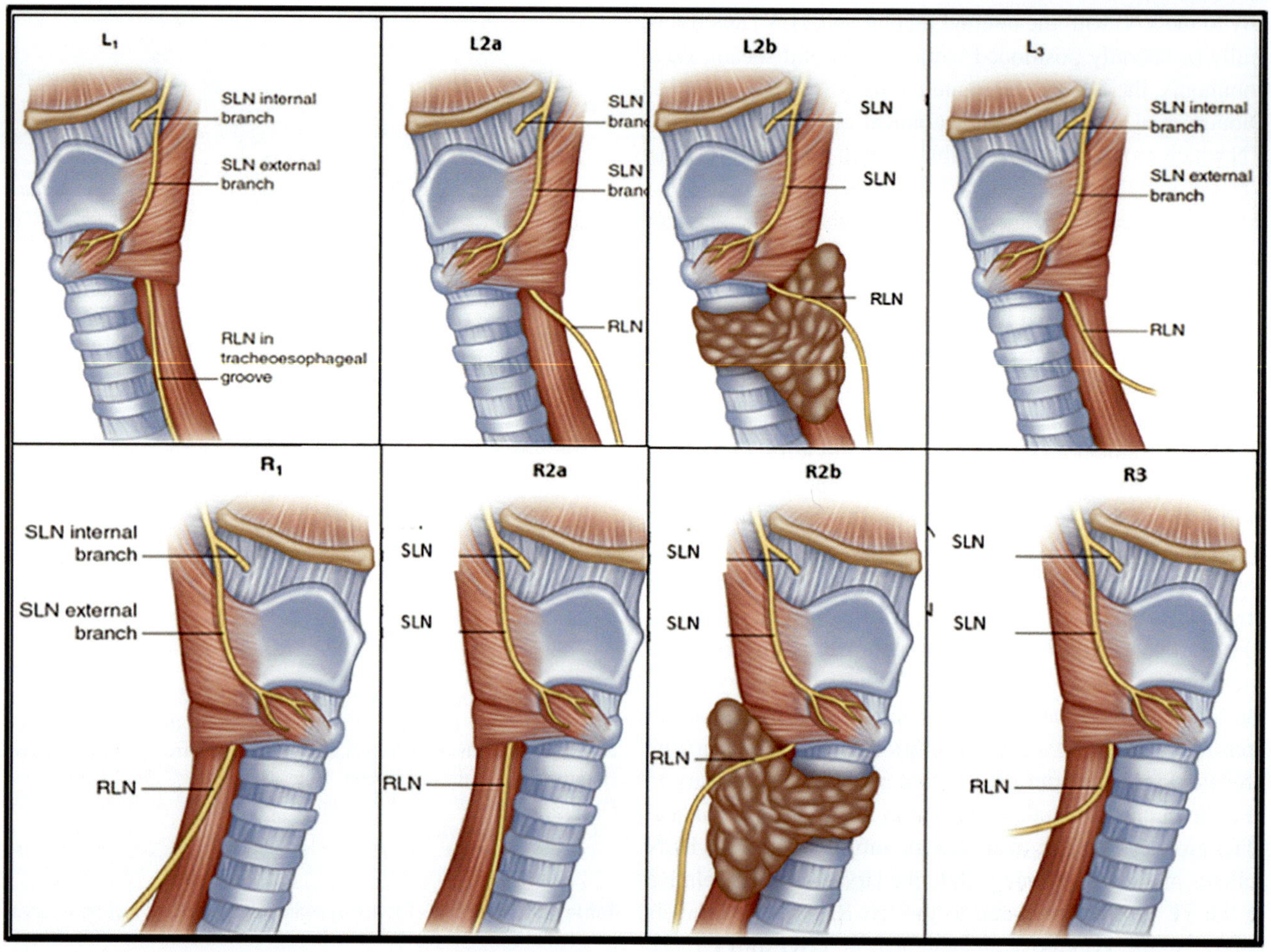


**Fig. 6.2** Basic classification of RLN surgical anatomic path in the neck base as it relates to the thyroid surgical procedure. *RLN* recurrent laryngeal nerve, *SLN* superior laryngeal nerve. (Adapted with permission from *The Recurrent and Superior Laryngeal Nerves*, Chapter 12, Randolph GW, Ed, copyright Springer Nature)

nificant surgical risk if not identified [63, 64]. On the right, the nonrecurrent RLN **(R3)** will not be found coursing under the inferior thyroid artery and instead will follow a more direct, medial course from the VN to the larynx without "recurring." This situation develops when the right subclavian artery arises from the distal aortic arch and extends in a retroesophageal course, which can be appreciated on preoperative imaging. A left nonrecurrent RLN **(L3)** is extremely rare, as a number of embryological anomalies, including situs inversus, aberrant subclavian artery, and ductus arteriosus, must occur in combination.

Extralaryngeal branching of the RLN occurs in up to 90% of subjects [57] with extralaryngeal branching of the primary motor fibers that contribute to an EMG response occurring in up to 25% [65]. This "true" extralaryngeal branching occurs near the ligament of Berry, below the border of the inferior constrictor muscle. The anterior motor branch is typically smaller in caliber than the posterior sensory branch and if not anticipated and identified can be inadvertently injured during dissection.

In a recent multicenter international study of 1000 nerves at risk during thyroid surgery, Liddy et al. found that nearly a quarter of nerves (23%) followed an abnormal intraoperative trajectory [66]. Loss of IONM signal was reported in 3.5% of cases overall and in 34% of cases where the RLN followed an unpredicted abnormal anatomic course. This degree of previously unreported significant anatomic variability of the RLN, which places the nerve at increased risk of injury, underscores the value of intraoperative nerve identification and mapping supplemented by dynamic functional assessment with IONM.

## Standard Set-up and Troubleshooting

### Standard Set-up

Effective use of IONM requires a basic appreciation for how neuromonitoring systems function. The fundamental components include stimulating and recording electrodes which are

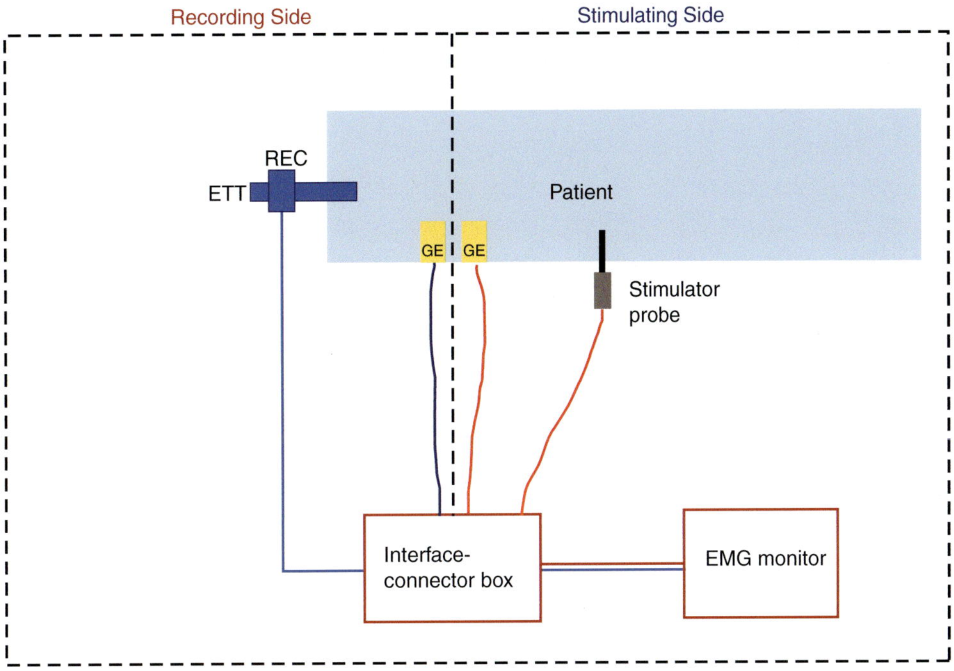


**Fig. 6.3** Schematic depicting the recording and stimulating sides of an intraoperative neuromonitoring system. *ETT* endotracheal tube, *REC* recording electrode, *GE* grounding electrode. (Adapted with permission from *Surgery of the Thyroid and Parathyroid Glands, 3rd Ed.* Chapter 36; fig. 36.13. Randolph, GW, Ed, copyright Elsevier)

integrated into a system that measures and displays evoked electromyography (EMG) waveforms. Monitoring systems are comprised of a recording side and a stimulating side (Fig. 6.3). The **recording side** contains the recording electrodes, grounding electrode (placed at the patient's shoulder), and a connector box which interfaces with the monitor. Needle-based or surface recording electrodes may be used. ETT-based systems with surface electrodes embedded in the ETT and placed at the level of the glottis are the preferred method because of their ease of set-up, noninvasive nature, and ability to easily record vocalis muscle EMG activity. Post-cricoid, trans-cartilaginous, or trans-cutaneous surface electrodes are additional options. Endoscopically placed intramuscular electrodes (hook wires) or electrodes placed through the cricothyroid membrane into the thyroarytenoid muscle have also been used.

The **stimulating side** contains the neural stimulating electrode, grounding electrode (placed at the shoulder), the connector-interface box, and a stimulation current pulse generator housed within the monitor. Stimulating probes may be unipolar, bipolar, or integrated into various dissecting instruments. Monopolar probes are most effective in eliciting neural stimulation through overlying tissue or fascia, which is especially useful during neural mapping. Bipolar electrodes provide a more focused stimulus with greater specificity but are less useful in neural mapping and require a higher stimulation current to elicit a maximal response. Stimulating instruments allow for simultaneous stimulation and dissection and are preferred by some surgeons. Continuous intraoperative neuromonitoring (CIONM) represents a relatively newer format of monitoring in which placement of a temporary vagal electrode provides automatic periodic stimulation (APS) of the vagus nerve to allow uninterrupted RLN monitoring. CIONM is addressed in greater detail in a later chapter.

Close collaboration with anesthesia providers is essential to safe and effective use of IONM. Long-acting neuromuscular blockade must be avoided in order to allow for detection of EMG activity. Use of lubricating ointments on the ETT should also be avoided. Pooling of saliva in the glottis can interfere with the function of the recording electrodes and should be managed with suction when necessary. Use of an anticholinergic drying agent may be helpful toward prevention of pooled secretions. At the time of initial intubation, the surgeon should be present to facilitate and confirm correct placement of the ETT with the electrodes situated at the level of the glottis. Displacement of the ETT may occur with positioning the patient into full neck extension, with translation as much as 2 cm into and 3 cm out of the airway after intubation in a neutral position [67]. Additionally, rotation of the ETT may occur, disrupting the extent of vocal cord contact with the recording electrodes. Confirmation of appropriate ETT placement should therefore occur after patient positioning. Use of a video-assisted laryngoscope may be especially helpful in visually confirming proper placement of the ETT (Fig. 6.4). Alternatively, respiratory variation may be observed on the neuromonitoring system, confirming contact of the recording electrodes with the glottis [68]. Respiratory variation appears as spontaneous saw-toothed shape waveforms between 30 and 70 μV (Fig. 6.5). This observation should take place after short-acting paralytic has worn off and before the patient enters a deep plane of anesthesia, timing which requires close collaboration and communication

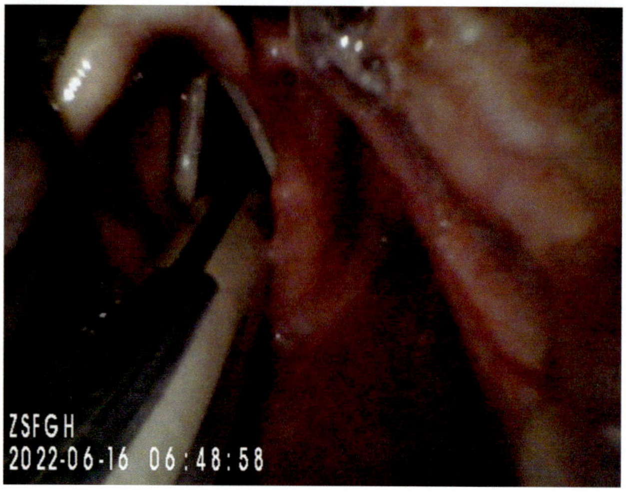


**Fig. 6.4** Use of videolaryngoscopy helps confirm proper positioning of the endotracheal tube surface electrodes with respect to the glottis

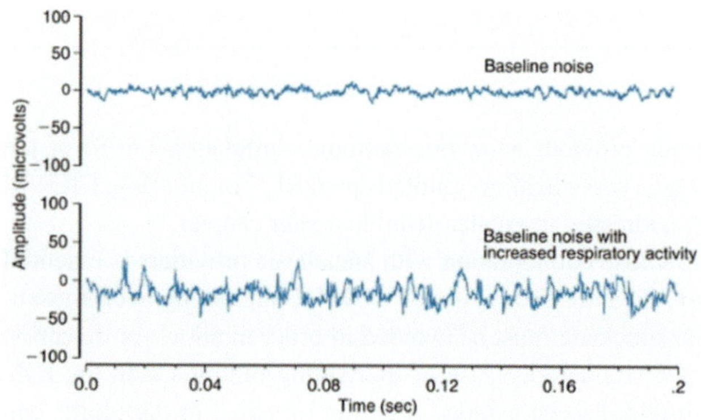


**Fig. 6.5** Baseline noise between 10 and 20 μV (upper line) and baseline noise with respiratory variation (bottom line), typically between 30 and 70 μV and characterized a saw-tooth pattern. (Reproduced with permission from *Surgery of the Thyroid and Parathyroid Glands, 3rd Ed.* Chapter 36; fig. 36.18 A. Randolph, GW, Ed, copyright Elsevier)

with anesthesia colleagues. The mechanical "tap test" produces waveforms which are poorly understood and likely represent artifact and is not recommended as method of confirming proper ETT placement [68].

After the ETT is confirmed to be in proper position, it is secured to the patient with note of its depth marking. Care should be taken to ensure the ventilatory circuit does not put undue weight or torque on the ETT, which can lead to unfavorable displacement or rotation of the ETT. Electrodes are connected to the connecting box-interface and impedance values are assessed. Low impedance values suggest good electrode contact with the vocal cords; each electrode should have an impedance value less than 5 k∧ with an imbalance between the two electrodes of less than 1 k∧ [69]. Large impedance imbalance may suggest incorrect ETT placement and should prompt repositioning. If the overall impedance is high, the ground electrodes should be checked or replaced. Once the set-up is complete, the monitor event threshold should be set at 100 μV and the stimulator probe set to a pulsatile output of 4 per second with a stimulating current of 1–2 mA. The electrocautery unit should be moved at least 10 feet away from the neuromonitoring unit to avoid interference.

## Signal Interpretation and Troubleshooting

Effective utilization of neuromonitoring information during surgical procedures requires a basic understanding of the electrophysiologic properties of EMG waveforms. When an electrical stimulus is applied to a motor nerve, the resulting muscle depolarization produces a biphasic waveform that is described in terms of its amplitude and latency. *Amplitude* is defined as the distance spanning the lowest to the highest point on the wave and correlates with the number of muscle fibers activated during the stimulus. *Latency* is defined as the time between the stimulus and the peak of the biphasic waveform and reflects the speed or ease of stimulation as well as the distance the stimulus travels. Normative values for latency and amplitude have been established for the left and right VN, RLN, and EBSLN and are shown in Fig. 6.6. Amplitudes may vary widely within and between subjects, likely due to a variety of factors, including the degree of contact with the probe and/or electrodes, patient factors which contribute to the size and number of activating muscle fibers such as age and sex, and local factors such as amount of overlying tissue and moisture and temperature levels [70]. The left VN is associated with a higher latency than the right because the left RLN assumes a longer course as it loops beneath the aortic arch before returning to the neck. A greater amplitude has also been noted for the right compared to the left VN [71].

During neuromonitored procedures, observation of a biphasic waveform indicates a veritable EMG response, distinguishable from artifact which appears on the monitor as disorganized electrical activity and can be produced by metal-on-metal contact or manipulation of the endotracheal tube (ETT) within the airway. The level of current which first triggers a recognizable EMG waveform response is termed *threshold*. For the VN and RLN, the threshold is typically 0.3 mA. Caragacianu et al. demonstrated no difference in amplitude when the nerve is stimulated by suprathreshold levels of 1 vs. 2 mA [72]. Stimulation at 1– 2 mA is physiologically similar to spontaneous vocal cord depolarization, as occurs during phonation, and is recommended by the INSMG for use as the stimulating current during neuromonitored thyroid and parathyroid procedures [7, 73].

To avoid inaccuracies in signal interpretation, the surgeon must be familiar with various prognostic testing errors. Loss of EMG signal (LOS, defined by the INMSG as an amplitude of <100 μV [7]) at the end of surgery is considered a positive test (associated with RLN paralysis), whereas maintenance

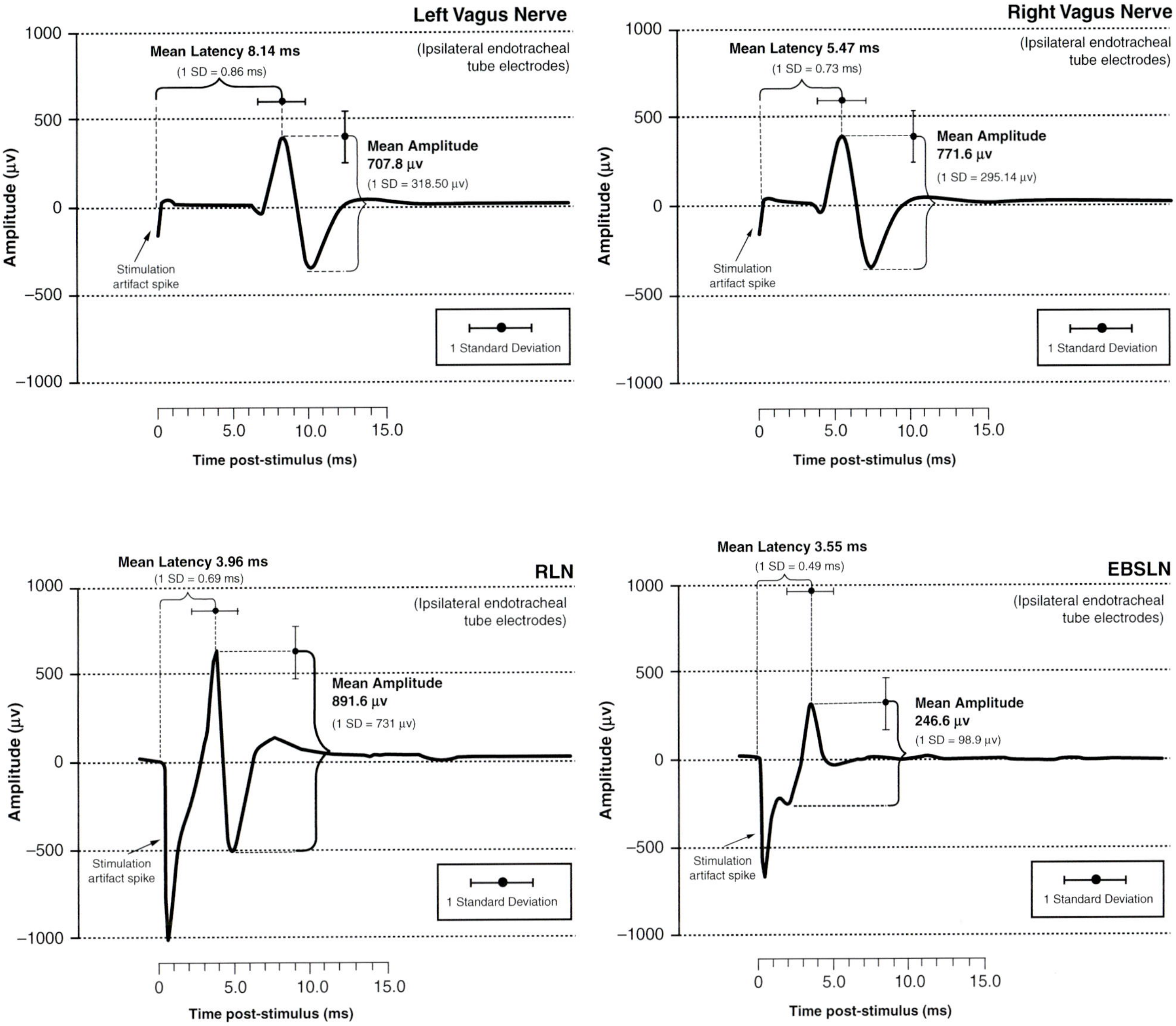


**Fig. 6.6** Normative EMG summated data, including mean amplitude and latency values for stimulated right and left vagus nerves, RLN and EBSLN. *EMG* electromyographic, *RLN* recurrent laryngeal nerve, *EBSLN* external branch of the superior laryngeal nerve, *SD* standard deviation. (Reproduced with permission from *Surgery of the Thyroid and Parathyroid Glands, 3rd Ed.* Chapter 36; fig. 36.26. Randolph, GW, Ed, copyright Elsevier)

of EMG activity is considered a negative test. There are several causes of false-positive tests (LOS with intact vocal cord mobility postoperatively). These include ETT malposition (most common), inadequate stimulus or failure of stimulus conduction due to overlying blood or fascia, use of neuromuscular blockade, and early neural recovery after injury. False negative tests (maintenance of EMG signal with postoperative VCP) may occur due to stimulation being applied distal to an injured segment, injury occurring after the last stimulus is applied (as when obtaining hemostasis), and evolving neural injury which develops after surgery is completed.

At the initiation of surgery, stimulation of strap muscles with observation of a gross muscle twitch confirms the absence of neuromuscular blockade and verifies the circuit is intact. Subsequently, dissection and stimulation of the ipsilateral VN should be performed to confirm a positive response on the neuromonitoring system. Stimulation of the VN can be accomplished by placing a stimulation probe set to 2–3 mA directly on the carotid sheath or VN to verify RLN function and working circuit [74]. This allows RLN mapping and dissection to proceed safely [47]. Without a positive response, a negative response cannot be accepted as a true negative. The INMSG recommends that stimulation of the VN (V1) with 1–2 mA produce an initial baseline response of >500 µV along with a detectable laryngeal twitch [7]. Appreciation of the laryngeal twitch is accomplished by placing a finger on the posterior aspect of the cricoid cartilage in order to palpate contraction of the posterior cricoarytenoid muscle during VN or RLN stimulation.

If LOS occurs and an equipment-associated error is suspected, laryngeal twitch should be assessed as a first step. Presence of an intact twitch indicates the stimulating side of the system is functional and a recording side error should be considered. Electrical connections and grounding electrodes should be checked, and the position of the ETT should be assessed. The anesthesia provider can be asked to rotate, insert, or withdraw the ETT during neural stimulation to assess whether signal returns. Conversely, if LOS occurs and laryngeal twitch is absent, a stimulating side error should be considered. Stimulation in a dry field and testing the probe on muscle can confirm adequate stimulating current and absence of neuromuscular blocking agents. If a stimulating problem is not detected, stimulation of the contralateral VN should be performed. If the contralateral VN response is present, an ipsilateral neural injury should be considered.

## RLN Injury and Loss of Signal

### Mechanisms of RLN Injury

Intraoperative RLN injury may occur from a variety of mechanisms, including stretch, compression, thermal injury, or transection. In a series of 281 injured RLNs, Dionigi et al. found traction injury was most common (71%), followed by thermal (17%), compression (4.2%), clamping (3.4%), ligature entrapment (1.6%), suction (1.4%), and transection (1.4%) [75]. Traction injuries occur most commonly at the Ligament of Berry where dense fibrous tissue may tether the nerve and cause it to stretch upon manipulation of the thyroid gland [6, 59, 76]. Importantly, traction injuries are not associated with visible evidence of damage, emphasizing the importance of neuromonitoring for functional assessment.

### Loss of Signal

LOS may occur as a segmental injury (type 1) in which there is complete loss of response proximal to the injured segment but preservation of neural stimulation distal to it. Retrograde stimulation of the nerve can be used to map out the neuropraxic segment and may be used to elucidate the mechanism of injury through review of any factors contributing to excessive tension, compression, or other forms of injury. LOS may also occur as a global-type injury (type 2) where there is complete loss of signal along the entire course of the VN and RLN without an identifiable point of injury. The etiology of type 2 injuries is not well-understood though is suspected to be related to intra-laryngeal dysfunction [47]. In a multi-institutional study, Schneider et al. prospectively examined 115 LOS cases and found traction to be the causative mechanism in 68% of type 1 injuries and 92% of type 2 injuries [76]. In this series, rates of permanent VCP were higher in type 1 LOS, though in a recent study of 1000 nerves at risk with 35 cases of LOS, Liddy et al. found poorer long-term recovery for type 2 cases [66, 76].

As previously noted, an important application of IONM involves the detection of adverse EMG changes which signal impending development of neuropraxia. During neuromonitored procedures, attention is paid to changes in amplitude and latency from baseline levels as surgical maneuvers are performed. A change characterized by a concordant amplitude decrease of >50% and latency increase of >10% suggests impending development of neuropraxia and should direct the surgeon to cease the associated maneuver [58]. It should be noted that frequent passive EMG activity occurring without stimulation may imply mechanical nerve injury or cautery stress and should similarly prompt assessment of the surgical maneuver associated with the activity. Several researchers have correlated such bursts of passive activity with some degree of nerve injury [77–79], but direct correlation with VCP has not been demonstrated.

When performing surgical maneuvers that especially place the RLN at risk of injury, frequent and repeated stimulation of the VN or RLN may be performed to monitor for adverse EMG changes. Alternatively, use of CIONM (discussed in a later chapter) allows for uninterrupted monitoring during high-risk maneuvers, potentially allowing the surgeon to modify or abort an injurious maneuver before a significant adverse EMG event occurs. Importantly, adverse EMG changes reverse in approximately 70–80% of cases if the injurious surgical maneuver is aborted or modified within 40–60 s. However, if repeated adverse events occur, EMG changes become less reversible with and there is increased risk of loss of LOS [7, 58, 59].

LOS is associated with a high likelihood of neuropraxia (positive predictive value of 83%) with only a 17–25% likelihood of intraoperative recovery. In order to maximize the predictive value of signal recovery, the INMSG has proposed that recovery be defined as a return of signal to >50% of the initial baseline amplitude, with a minimum absolute value of 250 μV. This coincides with 50% of the recommended minimum response of 500 μV for initial vagal stimulation [7]. When recovery occurs, it typically takes place within 20 min [80, 81]. If signal recovery occurs, the contralateral surgery can proceed. However, if LOS persists after waiting period of 20 min, staging of contralateral surgery should be considered to avoid risk of bilateral VCP [7].

When contemplating staged surgery, the INMSG recommends that the surgeon acknowledges the morbidity of bilateral VCP and tracheotomy and prioritizes this over concerns about altering the original plan [7]. Goretzki et al. reported that if surgery proceeded to the contralateral side with a known or unrecognized paresis on the first side, the risk of bilateral VCP was 17% [82]. The high level of risk may be attributable to patient-related factors, including bilaterally symmetric high-risk anatomic variants. Surgeon-related factors such as increased stress and its impact on surgical dexterity, cognition, and decision-making may also play a role [83]. The concept of staged surgery after LOS has gained acceptance in the surgical community. Dralle et al. evaluated willingness to stage surgery after LOS in a survey distributed to over 1200 surgical departments in Germany, with 94% of respondents indicating they would change their surgical plan in this setting [20].

In some cases, and particularly in the setting of surgery for thyroid cancer, a decision may be made to proceed to the contralateral side after LOS. This type of decision should take into account multiple factors, including the mechanism of neural injury, the likelihood and expected timing of neural recovery, degree of disease aggressivity, and the urgency and necessity of complete thyroidectomy. The patient's fitness for and willingness to undergo a second anesthesia should also be considered. Importantly, a preoperative dialogue with the patient and a multidisciplinary treatment team is important to streamline intraoperative decision-making, manage patient expectations, and facilitate informed consent.

For each patient, documentation of preoperative laryngeal examination (L1) followed by initial intraoperative supra-threshold vagus stimulation (V1) and RLN stimulation (R1) should be performed. At the conclusion of surgery, this data should be mirrored by documentation of final intraoperative RLN stimulation (R2), vagus stimulation (V2), and postoperative laryngeal examination (L2).

## IONM and RLN Invasion

Knowledge of preoperative vocal cord function is imperative for optimal decision-making in surgical management of the invaded nerve, especially as it relates to application of IONM. Preoperative VCP is an excellent predictor of RLN invasion, noted to be present in 70% of patients with invasive thyroid cancer compared with 0.3% in benign or noninvasive disease [39]. However, because nearly a third of patients with unilateral VCP are asymptomatic and produce a normal voice, reliance on voice abnormality as a marker for VCP is problematic and preoperative laryngeal examination should be performed [39–41].

A primary decision point in management of the invaded nerve involves whether the nerve should be preserved or resected. Preoperative laryngeal function and neuromonitoring information figure prominently into this decision, as do the patient's age, disease characteristics, overall health status, and preferences. Part II of the INSMG guidelines extensively details the patient- and disease-related factors which should be considered for optimal intraoperative decision-making [56].

When preoperative laryngeal function is intact, attempts should be made to preserve the RLN through shave excision, provided this is technically feasible and consistent with the overall therapeutic goals of surgery. While LOS may occur with this maneuver, neural function has been shown to recover majority of cases [84, 85]. When preoperative VCP is present, neuromonitoring information informs the decision of whether to preserve or resect the RLN through assessment of proximal stimulability. Kamani et al. demonstrated that 33% of invaded nerves with preoperative laryngeal dysfunction maintain the ability to generate an EMG response when stimulated proximal to the point of invasion [86]. It is assumed that some baseline level of neural transmission is maintained such that resection of the nerve then leads to loss of muscle tone and worsening of laryngeal function. Chi et al. demonstrated that preservation of invaded nerves with preoperative VCP but intact proximal stimulability prevents development of vocal cord atrophy and decline of vocal function [87]. The INMSG recommends that proximal stimulability be used as a parameter for decision-making in this setting [56].

Algorithms for management of the invaded RLN utilizing neuromonitoring information are published by the INMSG [56]. These algorithms are based on preoperative vocal cord status and can be summarized as the following:

1. Invaded nerve with normal preoperative vocal cord function

   When preoperative laryngoscopy is normal, extent of neural involvement guides the decision to preserve or resect the nerve, with shave resection being recommended for superficial involvement. Patient- and disease-related factors, including age, disease aggressiveness, and expected efficacy of adjuvant treatment, guide decision-making for more extensive neural involvement. To reduce the risk of bilateral VCP in planned bilateral surgery when neural resection is judged to be indicated, the INMSG recommends dissection be halted before LOS and surgery proceed to the contralateral side. If LOS occurs on the contralateral side, staged surgery may be offered to allow for neural recovery. If LOS does not occur, resection of the invaded ipsilateral nerve can be safely undertaken if indicated.
2. Invaded nerve with preoperative ipsilateral VCP

   When preoperative ipsilateral VCP is present, the INMSG recommends dissection of the contralateral side proceed first. Any contralateral signal abnormalities may then recover over the duration of the remaining surgical procedure. Moreover, when function of the contralateral nerve is known to be preserved, testing of proximal stimulability for the ipsilateral invaded nerve may then be used to direct management of the invaded nerve. In the absence of proximal stimulability, the invaded nerve is resected. If proximal stimulability is intact, patient- and disease-related factors guide decision-making.

3. Invaded only-functioning nerve (Contralateral VCP)

   In cases where pre-existing contralateral VCP is present and surgery of an invaded but only-functioning nerve is undertaken, careful shave excision with adjuvant treatment is recommended. Resection followed by tracheotomy for bilateral VCP should be reserved for rare cases.

## Neuromonitoring in Parathyroid Surgery

While parathyroidectomy does not routinely require identification or dissection of the RLN, the proximity of the parathyroid glands to the RLN poses risk of neural injury. Knowledge of the parathyroid gland anatomy relative to the position of the RLN is imperative for safe surgery. The superior parathyroid glands develop from the fourth branchial pouch and migrate a relatively short distance to their final position, which is most commonly on the posterior aspect of the thyroid gland near the cricothyroid joint. The superior glands lie dorsal to the RLN. By contrast, the inferior parathyroid glands develop from the third branchial pouch, travel with the thymus, and have a relatively longer and more variable path of migration inferiorly. The inferior parathyroid glands may be located at the level of the inferior thyroid lobe on the anterior or posterolateral surface, along the thyrothymic ligament or within thymic tongue in the upper mediastinum. The inferior parathyroid glands are situated ventral to the RLN.

Identification of an enlarged parathyroid gland as inferior or superior in origin has important bearing on surgical approach as it relates to management of the RLN. In particular, enlarged superior parathyroid glands may descend over time into the upper mediastinum, a process attributed to gravity, favorable tissue planes, and swallowing movements [88]. Importantly, these overly descended superior glands retain their dorsal relationship to the RLN. An enlarged gland which appears inferior to the thyroid but is situated in a deep dorsal position should prompt consideration of an overly descended superior gland. Failure to recognize the superior origin of gland may lead to inadvertent RLN injury upon removal. Neuromonitoring may be especially useful in this context to map the course of the RLN and confirm its location relative to the enlarged parathyroid gland.

While neuromonitoring is recognized as an invaluable tool in thyroid surgery, its application to parathyroid surgery has been less well-examined. Most studies address IONM in both thyroid and parathyroid surgery. A single study performed by Mourad et al. investigated outcomes for parathyroid surgery alone. This group retrospectively studied 213 patients who underwent parathyroidectomy, 87 of whom were in the historical cohort that did not undergo neuromonitored surgery. These authors found a 4.5% rate of postoperative VCP in the unmonitored group, compared with a 4% rate of VCP in the neuromonitored group, a difference which did not meet statistical significance. Notably, of the 5 RLN injuries which occurred in the neuromonitored group of 126 patients, 3 were in reoperative cases [89]. These findings highlight the complex and challenging nature of reoperative parathyroid surgery, where scar and altered anatomy may pose challenges to nerve preservation. In reoperative cases, and in patients who have undergone prior thyroidectomy, IONM may be especially helpful in facilitating neural mapping and identification.

Neuromonitoring has special significance for bilateral parathyroid exploration in which both RLNs are placed at risk. While focused surgery has fallen into favor for treatment of single adenomas, a bilateral approach may be indicated for multigland or non-localizing disease. In this context, confirmation of intact RLN function on the initially operated side is prudent prior to progressing to the contralateral side in order to avoid risk of bilateral VCP.

## Conclusions

RLN preservation during thyroid and parathyroid surgery is an important and complex task. Knowledge of RLN anatomy and sound surgical skills are critical to this effort. As an adjunctive tool, IONM has several applications which facilitate successful nerve identification and preservation. Effective utilization of IONM requires knowledge of equipment functionality in order to avoid pitfalls associated with equipment errors. Standards of use proposed by the INMSG support optimal utilization of IONM and facilitate further study of its benefit.

## References

1. Kaplan EL, Salti GI, Roncella M, Fulton N, Kadowaki M. History of the recurrent laryngeal nerve: from Galen to Lahey. World J Surg. 2009;33(3):386–93.
2. Dralle H, Sekulla C, Haerting J, Timmermann W, Neumann HJ, Kruse E, et al. Risk factors of paralysis and functional outcome after recurrent laryngeal nerve monitoring in thyroid surgery. Surgery. 2004;136(6):1310–22.
3. Lahey FH, Hoover WB. Injuries to the recurrent laryngeal nerve in thyroid operations: their management and avoidance. Ann Surg. 1938;108(4):545–62.
4. Riddell VH. Injury to recurrent laryngeal nerves during thyroidectomy, a comparison between the results of identification and non-identification in 1022 nerves exposed to risk. Lancet Lond Engl. 1956;271(6944):638–41.
5. Snyder SK, Lairmore TC, Hendricks JC, Roberts JW. Elucidating mechanisms of recurrent laryngeal nerve injury during thyroidectomy and parathyroidectomy. J Am Coll Surg. 2008;206(1):123–30.
6. Chiang FY, Lu IC, Kuo WR, Lee KW, Chang NC, Wu CW. The mechanism of recurrent laryngeal nerve injury during thyroid sur-

gery--the application of intraoperative neuromonitoring. Surgery. 2008;143(6):743–9.

7. Schneider R, Randolph GW, Dionigi G, Wu CW, Barczynski M, Chiang FY, et al. International neural monitoring study group guideline 2018 part I: staging bilateral thyroid surgery with monitoring loss of signal. Laryngoscope. 2018;128(Suppl 3):S1–17.
8. Shedd DP, Durham C. Electrical identification of the recurrent laryngeal nerve. I. Response of the canine larynx to electrical stimulation of the recurrent laryngeal nerve. Ann Surg. 1966;163(1):47–50.
9. Flisberg K, Lindholm T. Electrical stimulation of the human recurrent laryngeal nerve during thyroid operation. Acta Otolaryngol Suppl. 1969;263:63–7.
10. Riddell V. Thyroidectomy: prevention of bilateral recurrent nerve palsy. Results of identification of the nerve over 23 consecutive years (1946-69) with a description of an additional safety measure. Br J Surg. 1970;57(1):1–11.
11. Engel PM, Büter HA, Page PS, Mos A. A device for the location and protection of the recurrent laryngeal nerve during operations upon the neck. Surg Gynecol Obstet. 1981;152(6):825–6.
12. Gavilán J, Gavilán C. Recurrent laryngeal nerve. Identification during thyroid and parathyroid surgery. Arch Otolaryngol Head Neck Surg. 1986;112(12):1286–8.
13. James AG, Crocker S, Woltering E, Ferrara J, Farrar W. A simple method for identifying and testing the recurrent laryngeal nerve. Surg Gynecol Obstet. 1985;161(2):185–6.
14. Rice DH, Cone-Wesson B. Intraoperative recurrent laryngeal nerve monitoring. Otolaryngol Head Neck Surg. 1991;105(3):372–5.
15. Eisele DW. Intraoperative electrophysiologic monitoring of the recurrent laryngeal nerve. Laryngoscope. 1996;106(4):443–9.
16. Horne SK, Gal TJ, Brennan JA. Prevalence and patterns of intraoperative nerve monitoring for thyroidectomy. Otolaryngol Head Neck Surg. 2007;136(6):952–6.
17. Sturgeon C, Sturgeon T, Angelos P. Neuromonitoring in thyroid surgery: attitudes, usage patterns, and predictors of use among endocrine surgeons. World J Surg. 2009;33(3):417–25.
18. Marti JL, Holm T, Randolph G. Universal use of intraoperative nerve monitoring by recently fellowship-trained thyroid surgeons is common, associated with higher surgical volume, and impacts intraoperative decision-making. World J Surg. 2016;40(2):337–43.
19. Feng AL, Puram SV, Singer MC, Modi R, Kamani D, Randolph GW. Increased prevalence of neural monitoring during thyroidectomy: global surgical survey. Laryngoscope. 2020;130(4):1097–104.
20. Dralle H, Sekulla C, Lorenz K, Nguyen Thanh P, Schneider R, Machens A. Loss of the nerve monitoring signal during bilateral thyroid surgery. Br J Surg. 2012;99(8):1089–95.
21. Bartsch DK, Dotzenrath C, Vorländer C, Zielke A, Weber T, Buhr HJ, et al. Current practice of surgery for benign goitre-an analysis of the prospective DGAV StuDoQ|thyroid registry. J Clin Med. 2019;8(4):E477.
22. Ho Y, Carr MM, Goldenberg D. Trends in intraoperative neural monitoring for thyroid and parathyroid surgery amongst otolaryngologists and general surgeons. Eur Arch Otorhinolaryngol. 2013;270(9):2525–30.
23. Singer MC, Rosenfeld RM, Sundaram K. Laryngeal nerve monitoring: current utilization among head and neck surgeons. Otolaryngol Head Neck Surg. 2012;146(6):895–9.
24. Dionigi G, Bacuzzi A, Boni L, Rovera F, Dionigi R. What is the learning curve for intraoperative neuromonitoring in thyroid surgery? Int J Surg Lond Engl. 2008;6(Suppl 1):S7–12.
25. The American Academy of Otolaryngology. Head and neck surgery foundation [Internet]. Available from: www.OTOSOURCE.org.
26. The American Head and Neck Society (AHNS) [Internet]. Available from: www.ahns.info.
27. The American Association of Endocrine Surgeons. [Internet]. Available from: www.endocrinesurgery.org.
28. Wu CW, Randolph GW, Barczyński M, Schneider R, Chiang FY, Huang TY, et al. Training courses in laryngeal nerve monitoring in thyroid and parathyroid surgery- the INMSG consensus statement. Front Endocrinol. 2021;12:705346.
29. Hayward NJ, Grodski S, Yeung M, Johnson WR, Serpell J. Recurrent laryngeal nerve injury in thyroid surgery: a review. ANZ J Surg. 2013;83(1–2):15–21.
30. Jeannon JP, Orabi AA, Bruch GA, Abdalsalam HA, Simo R. Diagnosis of recurrent laryngeal nerve palsy after thyroidectomy: a systematic review. Int J Clin Pract. 2009;63(4):624–9.
31. Bergenfelz A, Jansson S, Kristoffersson A, Mårtensson H, Reihnér E, Wallin G, et al. Complications to thyroid surgery: results as reported in a database from a multicenter audit comprising 3,660 patients. Langenbeck's Arch Surg. 2008;393(5):667–73.
32. Nouraei SAR, Virk JS, Middleton SE, Aylin P, Mace A, Vaz F, et al. A national analysis of trends, outcomes and volume-outcome relationships in thyroid surgery. Clin Otolaryngol. 2017;42(2):354–65.
33. Sarkis LM, Zaidi N, Norlén O, Delbridge LW, Sywak MS, Sidhu SB. Bilateral recurrent laryngeal nerve injury in a specialized thyroid surgery unit: would routine intraoperative neuromonitoring alter outcomes? ANZ J Surg. 2017;87(5):364–7.
34. Jiang Y, Gao B, Zhang X, Zhao J, Chen J, Zhang S, et al. Prevention and treatment of recurrent laryngeal nerve injury in thyroid surgery. Int J Clin Exp Med. 2014;7(1):101–7.
35. Francis DO, Pearce EC, Ni S, Garrett CG, Penson DF. Epidemiology of vocal fold paralyses after total thyroidectomy for well-differentiated thyroid cancer in a Medicare population. Otolaryngol Head Neck Surg. 2014;150(4):548–57.
36. Dhillon VK, Randolph GW, Stack BC, Lindeman B, Bloom G, Sinclair CF, et al. Immediate and partial neural dysfunction after thyroid and parathyroid surgery: need for recognition, laryngeal exam, and early treatment. Head Neck. 2020;42(12):3779–94.
37. Wilson JA, Deary IJ, Millar A, Mackenzie K. The quality of life impact of dysphonia. Clin Otolaryngol Allied Sci. 2002;27(3):179–82.
38. Jones SM, Carding PN, Drinnan MJ. Exploring the relationship between severity of dysphonia and voice-related quality of life. Clin Otolaryngol. 2006;31(5):411–7.
39. Randolph GW, Kamani D. The importance of preoperative laryngoscopy in patients undergoing thyroidectomy: voice, vocal cord function, and the preoperative detection of invasive thyroid malignancy. Surgery. 2006;139(3):357–62.
40. Farrag TY, Samlan RA, Lin FR, Tufano RP. The utility of evaluating true vocal fold motion before thyroid surgery. Laryngoscope. 2006;116(2):235–8.
41. Brooks JA, Abdelhamid Ahmed AH, Al-Qurayshi Z, Kamani D. Recurrent laryngeal nerve invasion by thyroid cancer: laryngeal function and survival outcomes. Laryngoscope. 2022;132(11):2285–92.
42. Chandrasekhar SS, Randolph GW, Seidman MD, Rosenfeld RM, Angelos P, Barkmeier-Kraemer J, et al. Clinical practice guideline: improving voice outcomes after thyroid surgery. Otolaryngol Head Neck Surg. 2013;148(6 Suppl):S1–37.
43. Sinclair CF, Bumpous JM, Haugen BR, Chala A, Meltzer D, Miller BS, et al. Laryngeal examination in thyroid and parathyroid surgery: an American Head and Neck Society consensus statement: AHNS consensus statement. Head Neck. 2016;38(6):811–9.
44. Haugen BR, Alexander EK, Bible KC, Doherty GM, Mandel SJ, Nikiforov YE, et al. 2015 American Thyroid Association management guidelines for adult patients with thyroid nodules and differentiated thyroid cancer: the American Thyroid Association guidelines task force on thyroid nodules and differentiated thyroid cancer. Thyroid Off J Am Thyroid Assoc. 2016;26(1):1–133.
45. Shindo ML, Caruana SM, Kandil E, McCaffrey JC, Orloff LA, Porterfield JR, et al. Management of invasive well-differentiated

thyroid cancer: an American Head and Neck Society consensus statement. AHNS consensus statement. Head Neck. 2014;36(10):1379–90.
46. Musholt TJ, Clerici T, Dralle H, Frilling A, Goretzki PE, Hermann MM, et al. German Association of Endocrine Surgeons practice guidelines for the surgical treatment of benign thyroid disease. Langenbeck's Arch Surg. 2011;396(5):639–49.
47. Randolph GW, Dralle H, International Intraoperative Monitoring Study Group, Abdullah H, Barczynski M, Bellantone R, et al. Electrophysiologic recurrent laryngeal nerve monitoring during thyroid and parathyroid surgery: international standards guideline statement. Laryngoscope. 2011;121(Suppl 1):S1–16.
48. Zheng S, Xu Z, Wei Y, Zeng M, He J. Effect of intraoperative neuromonitoring on recurrent laryngeal nerve palsy rates after thyroid surgery--a meta-analysis. J Formos Med Assoc Taiwan Yi Zhi. 2013;112(8):463–72.
49. Higgins TS, Gupta R, Ketcham AS, Sataloff RT, Wadsworth JT, Sinacori JT. Recurrent laryngeal nerve monitoring versus identification alone on post-thyroidectomy true vocal fold palsy: a meta-analysis. Laryngoscope. 2011;121(5):1009–17.
50. Pisanu A, Porceddu G, Podda M, Cois A, Uccheddu A. Systematic review with meta-analysis of studies comparing intraoperative neuromonitoring of recurrent laryngeal nerves versus visualization alone during thyroidectomy. J Surg Res. 2014;188(1):152–61.
51. Yang S, Zhou L, Lu Z, Ma B, Ji Q, Wang Y. Systematic review with meta-analysis of intraoperative neuromonitoring during thyroidectomy. Int J Surg Lond Engl. 2017;39:104–13.
52. Staubitz JI, Watzka FM, Poplawski A. Effect of intraoperative nerve monitoring on postoperative vocal cord palsy rates after thyroidectomy: European multicentre registry-based study. BJS Open. 2020;4(5):821–9.
53. Wong KP, Mak KL, Wong CKH, Lang BHH. Systematic review and meta-analysis on intra-operative neuro-monitoring in high-risk thyroidectomy. Int J Surg Lond Engl. 2017;38:21–30.
54. Barczyński M, Konturek A, Pragacz K, Papier A, Stopa M, Nowak W. Intraoperative nerve monitoring can reduce prevalence of recurrent laryngeal nerve injury in thyroid reoperations: results of a retrospective cohort study. World J Surg. 2014;38(3):599–606.
55. Barczyński M, Konturek A, Cichoń S. Randomized clinical trial of visualization versus neuromonitoring of recurrent laryngeal nerves during thyroidectomy. Br J Surg. 2009;96(3):240–6.
56. Wu CW, Dionigi G, Barczynski M, Chiang FY, Dralle H, Schneider R, et al. International neuromonitoring study group guidelines 2018: part II: optimal recurrent laryngeal nerve management for invasive thyroid cancer-incorporation of surgical, laryngeal, and neural electrophysiologic data: INMSG loss of signal guidelines: part II. Laryngoscope. 2018;128:S18–27.
57. Fundakowski CE, Hales NW, Agrawal N, Barczyński M, Camacho PM, Hartl DM, et al. Surgical management of the recurrent laryngeal nerve in thyroidectomy: American head and neck society consensus statement. Head Neck. 2018;40(4):663–75.
58. Schneider R, Randolph GW, Sekulla C, Phelan E, Thanh PN, Bucher M, et al. Continuous intraoperative vagus nerve stimulation for identification of imminent recurrent laryngeal nerve injury. Head Neck. 2013;35(11):1591–8.
59. Phelan E, Schneider R, Lorenz K, Dralle H, Kamani D, Potenza A, et al. Continuous vagal IONM prevents recurrent laryngeal nerve paralysis by revealing initial EMG changes of impending neuropraxic injury: a prospective, multicenter study. Laryngoscope. 2014;124(6):1498–505.
60. Shoja MM, Ardalan MR, Tubbs RS, Loukas M, Vahedinia S, Jabbary R, et al. The relationship between the internal jugular vein and common carotid artery in the carotid sheath: the effects of age, gender and side. Ann Anat. 2008;190(4):339–43.
61. Dionigi G, Chiang FY, Rausei S, Wu CW, Boni L, Lee KW, et al. Surgical anatomy and neurophysiology of the vagus nerve (VN) for standardised intraoperative neuromonitoring (IONM) of the inferior laryngeal nerve (ILN) during thyroidectomy. Langenbeck's Arch Surg. 2010;395(7):893–9.
62. Randolph G, Wu C, Dionigi G, Kamani D, Modi R, Chiang F, et al. The international RLN anatomic classification system. In: Randolph GW, editor. The recurrent and superior laryngeal nerves. Springer; 2016. p. 125–38.
63. Kamani D, Potenza AS, Cernea CR, Kamani YV, Randolph GW. The nonrecurrent laryngeal nerve: anatomic and electrophysiologic algorithm for reliable identification. Laryngoscope. 2015;125(2):503–8.
64. Le VQ, Ngo QD, Ngo XQ. Nonrecurrent laryngeal nerve in thyroid surgery: frequency, anatomical variations according to a new classification and surgery consideration. Head Neck. 2019;41(9):2969–75.
65. Serpell J, Yeung M, Grodski S. The motor fibers of the recurrent laryngeal nerve are located in the anterior extralaryngeal branch. Ann Surg. 2009;249(4):648–52.
66. Liddy W, Wu CW, Dionigi G, Donatini G, Giles Senyurek Y, Kamani D, et al. Varied recurrent laryngeal nerve course is associated with increased risk of nerve dysfunction during thyroidectomy: results of the surgical anatomy of the recurrent laryngeal nerve in thyroid surgery study, an international multicenter prospective anatomic and electrophysiologic study of 1000 monitored nerves at risk from the International Neural Monitoring Study Group. Thyroid Off J Am Thyroid Assoc. 2021;31(11):1730–40.
67. Yap SJ, Morris RW, Pybus DA. Alterations in endotracheal tube position during general anaesthesia. Anaesth Intensive Care. 1994;22(5):586–8.
68. Chambers KJ, Pearse A, Coveney J, Rogers S, Kamani D, Sritharan N, et al. Respiratory variation predicts optimal endotracheal tube placement for intra-operative nerve monitoring in thyroid and parathyroid surgery. World J Surg. 2015;39(2):393–9.
69. Kamani D, Soylu S, Randolph GW. Neuromonitoring in thyroid surgery. In: Parameswaran R, Agarwal A, editors. Evidence-based endocrine surgery. Springer; 2018. p. 173–86.
70. Dabekaussen KFAA, Mallur P, Shin JJ. Basic and advanced electrophysiology, setup, and anesthesia. In: Scharpf J, Randolph GW, editors. Intraoperative cranial nerve monitoring in otolaryngology-head and neck surgery. Cham: Springer; 2022. p. 19–24.
71. Lorenz K, Sekulla C, Schelle J, Schmeiss B, Brauckhoff M, Dralle H, et al. What are normal quantitative parameters of intraoperative neuromonitoring (IONM) in thyroid surgery? Langenbeck's Arch Surg. 2010;395(7):901–9.
72. Caragacianu D, Kamani D, Randolph GW. Intraoperative monitoring: normative range associated with normal postoperative glottic function. Laryngoscope. 2013;123(12):3026–31.
73. Rodriquez AA, Myers BR, Ford CN. Laryngeal electromyography in the diagnosis of laryngeal nerve injuries. Arch Phys Med Rehabil. 1990;71(8):587–90.
74. Wu CW, Dionigi G, Chen HC, Chen HY, Lee KW, Lu IC, et al. Vagal nerve stimulation without dissecting the carotid sheath during intraoperative neuromonitoring of the recurrent laryngeal nerve in thyroid surgery. Head Neck. 2013;35(10):1443–7.
75. Dionigi G, Wu CW, Kim HY, Rausei S, Boni L, Chiang FY. Severity of recurrent laryngeal nerve injuries in thyroid surgery. World J Surg. 2016;40(6):1373–81.
76. Schneider R, Randolph G, Dionigi G, Barczyński M, Chiang FY, Triponez F, et al. Prospective study of vocal fold function after loss of the neuromonitoring signal in thyroid surgery: the International Neural Monitoring Study Group's POLT study. Laryngoscope. 2016;126(5):1260–6.

77. Dong CCJ, Macdonald DB, Akagami R, Westerberg B, Alkhani A, Kanaan I, et al. Intraoperative facial motor evoked potential monitoring with transcranial electrical stimulation during skull base surgery. Clin Neurophysiol. 2005;116(3):588–96.
78. Prass RL. Iatrogenic facial nerve injury: the role of facial nerve monitoring. Otolaryngol Clin N Am. 1996;29(2):265–75.
79. Pearlman RC, Isley MR, Ruben GD, Sandler SC, Weisbaum B, Khan MA, et al. Intraoperative monitoring of the recurrent laryngeal nerve using acoustic, free-run, and evoked electromyography. J Clin Neurophysiol. 2005;22(2):148–52.
80. Sitges-Serra A, Fontané J, Dueñas JP, Duque CS, Lorente L, Trillo L, et al. Prospective study on loss of signal on the first side during neuromonitoring of the recurrent laryngeal nerve in total thyroidectomy. Br J Surg. 2013;100(5):662–6.
81. Schneider R, Sekulla C, Machens A, Lorenz K, Thanh PN, Dralle H. Dynamics of loss and recovery of the nerve monitoring signal during thyroidectomy predict early postoperative vocal fold function. Head Neck. 2016;38(Suppl 1):E1144–51.
82. Goretzki PE, Schwarz K, Brinkmann J, Wirowski D, Lammers BJ. The impact of intraoperative neuromonitoring (IONM) on surgical strategy in bilateral thyroid diseases: is it worth the effort? World J Surg. 2010;34(6):1274–84.
83. Arora S, Sevdalis N, Nestel D, Tierney T, Woloshynowych M, Kneebone R. Managing intraoperative stress: what do surgeons want from a crisis training program? Am J Surg. 2009;197(4):537–43.
84. Lang BHH, Lo CY, Wong KP, Wan KY. Should an involved but functioning recurrent laryngeal nerve be shaved or resected in a locally advanced papillary thyroid carcinoma? Ann Surg Oncol. 2013;20(9):2951–7.
85. Kihara M, Miyauchi A, Yabuta T, Higashiyama T, Fukushima M, Ito Y, et al. Outcome of vocal cord function after partial layer resection of the recurrent laryngeal nerve in patients with invasive papillary thyroid cancer. Surgery. 2014;155(1):184–9.
86. Kamani D, Darr EA, Randolph GW. Electrophysiologic monitoring characteristics of the recurrent laryngeal nerve preoperatively paralyzed or invaded with malignancy. Otolaryngol Head Neck Surg. 2013;149(5):682–8.
87. Chi SY, Lammers B, Boehner H, Pohl P, Goretzki PE. Is it meaningful to preserve a palsied recurrent laryngeal nerve? Thyroid. 2008;18(3):363–6.
88. Thompson NW, Eckhauser FE, Harness JK. The anatomy of primary hyperparathyroidism. Surgery. 1982;92(5):814–21.
89. Mourad M, Kadakia S, Jategaonkar A, Gordin E, Ducic Y. Intraoperative nerve monitoring during parathyroid surgery: the Fort Worth experience. Head Neck. 2017;39(8):1662–4.

# 7 External Branch of the Superior Laryngeal Nerve (EBSLN) Monitoring During Thyroid and Parathyroid Surgery

Marcin Barczyński and Claudio R. Cernea

## Introduction

The EBSLN is a branch of the superior laryngeal nerve, which originates from the X cranial nerve [1]. It is the motor nerve of the CTM (Fig. 7.1). This muscle approximates the cricoid and the thyroid cartilage, stretching the vocal fold and increasing its tension, performing an opponent action to the thyroarytenoid muscle. This lengthening and tensioning of the vocal fold are essential for the production of high-frequency sounds, especially among female individuals and voice professionals.

## Surgical Anatomy

Many authors proposed several anatomical classifications for the relationship of EBSLN with the superior pedicle and the upper pole of the thyroid gland and the CTM. However, the most widely accepted and employed is the Cernea classification used in this chapter [3].

The EBSLN crosses the superior thyroid vessels on its way to the CTM, usually more than 1cm above the upper border of the superior thyroid pole. However, in about 14% [4] to 20% [5] of the situations, this crossing may happen well below the upper border of the superior thyroid pole. This is the type 2b EBSLN, according to the classification proposed by Cernea et al. [6] (Fig. 7.2). Clearly, this anatomical relationship increases the risk of nerve injury during ligation and cutting of the superior thyroid vessels (Fig. 7.3).

M. Barczyński (✉)
Department of Endocrine Surgery, Third Chair of General Surgery, Jagiellonian University Medical College, Krakow, Poland
e-mail: marcin.barczynski@uj.edu.pl

C. R. Cernea
Department of Surgery, University of São Paulo School of Medicine, São Paulo, São Paulo, Brazil

## How to Avoid Injury to the EBSLN During Thyroidectomy

The surgeon must exert caution when dissecting the superior thyroid pole, in order to avoid inadvertent injury of the EBSLN. It is important to emphasize that, even with the use of magnifying loupes (strongly advisable), it may be quite difficult to identify this nerve, which is usually much thinner than the inferior laryngeal nerve. The distal portion of the EBSLN frequently enters the CTM within the limits of the sternothyroid-laryngeal triangle, described by Moosman and DeWeese [7]. However, from the surgical point of view, it is more important to be able to identify the EBSLN at the area of the superior thyroid pole.

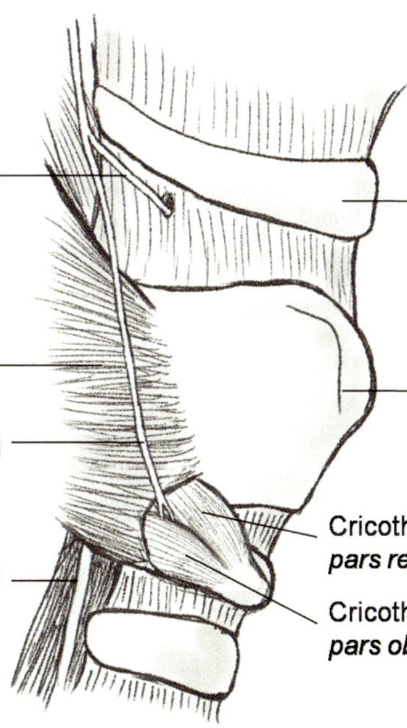


**Fig. 7.1** EBSLN descends dorsolaterally to carotid vessels, then crosses them medially, routing to the larynx (from Barczynski et al. [2]; with permission)


A. L. Shifrin et al. (eds.), *Atlas of Intraoperative Cranial Nerve Monitoring in Thyroid and Head and Neck Surgery*,
https://doi.org/10.1007/978-3-031-24613-5_7

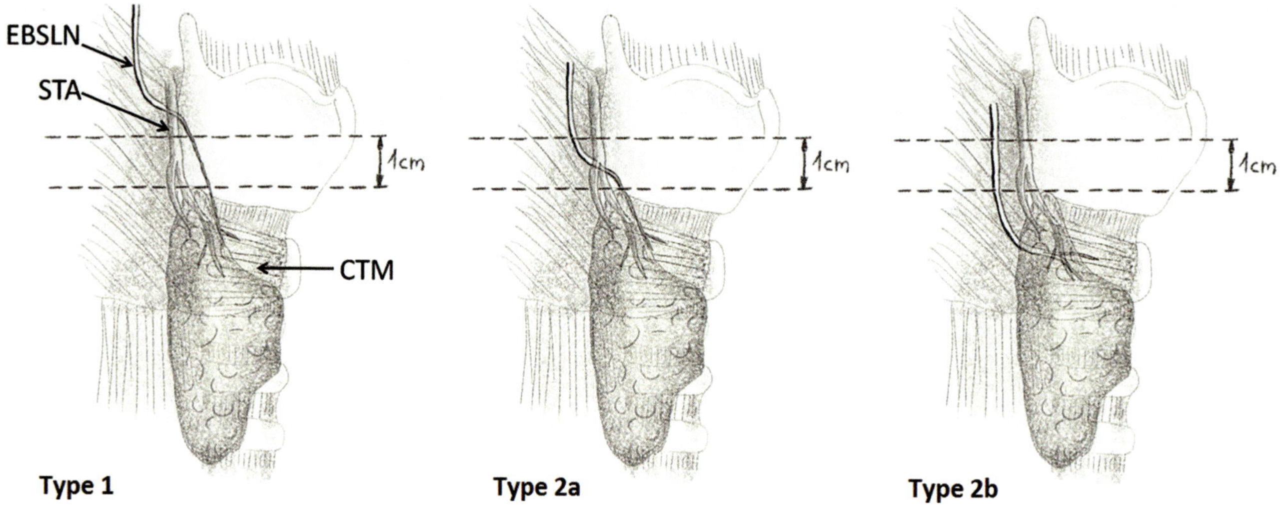


**Fig. 7.2** Cernea's external branch of the superior laryngeal nerve (EBSLN) surgical anatomic classification (from Barczynski et al. [2]; with permission)

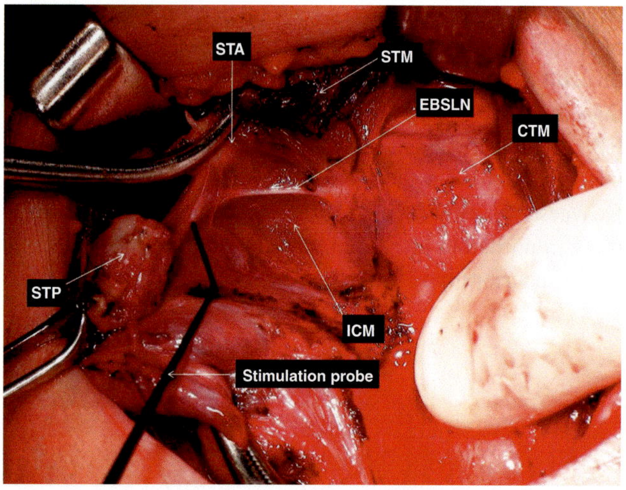


**Fig. 7.3** Meticulous dissection and ligation of individual branches of the superior thyroid artery with visual identification and electric stimulation of the EBSLN to assure functional preservation of the nerve. *EBSLN* external branch of the superior laryngeal nerve, *CTM* cricothyroid muscle, *ICM* inferior constrictor muscle, *STM* sternothyroid muscle, *STA* superior thyroid artery, *STP* superior thyroid pole

## How to Diagnose the EBSLN Paralysis?

In male individuals, the symptoms of EBSLN paralysis may be mild. However, in female patients and in voice professionals, usually there are symptomatic voice changes: vocal fatigue, difficulty to phonate in high-frequency tones, and lowering of the vocal register. Even at laryngoscopy, it may be quite difficult to detect this paralysis, as the features are far subtler than those that accompany paralysis of the inferior laryngeal nerve. The more common signs of EBSLN paralysis are: discrete bowing of the affected vocal fold, posterior glottic rotation toward the side of the paralysis, inferior displacement of the affected vocal fold, and asymmetry of the vocal fold mucosal wave [8]. When an injury of the EBSLN occurs, several parameters of the phonation may be affected: lowering of the voice register and difficulty for the production of acute sounds like "e" are the most usual consequences. The gold standard for the diagnosis of an EBSLN paralysis is the percutaneous electromyography of the CTM [5].

## Intraoperative Monitoring of the EBSLN

### Relevance of EBSLN Intraoperative Monitoring

During dissection of the superior thyroid pole, the identification of the EBSLN without any kind of magnification can be rather difficult. In fact, it has been reported that only one-third of the nerves can be positively identified in this way [2]. Thus, according to the recommendations of the guideline of the International Neural Monitoring Study Group, the surgeon is advised to use some form of nerve stimulation in order to enhance his or her capability to effectively identify the EBSLN (Fig. 7.4) [2]. The mnemonic formula shown in Fig. 7.5 summarizes surgical steps helpful in EBSLN identification with intraoperative nerve stimulation.

### Does EBSLN Intraoperative Monitoring Reduce the Frequency of Nerve Injury?

There are some reports in the literature suggesting that it is advisable to use intraoperative nerve monitoring of the EBSLN during dissection of the superior pole of the thyroid

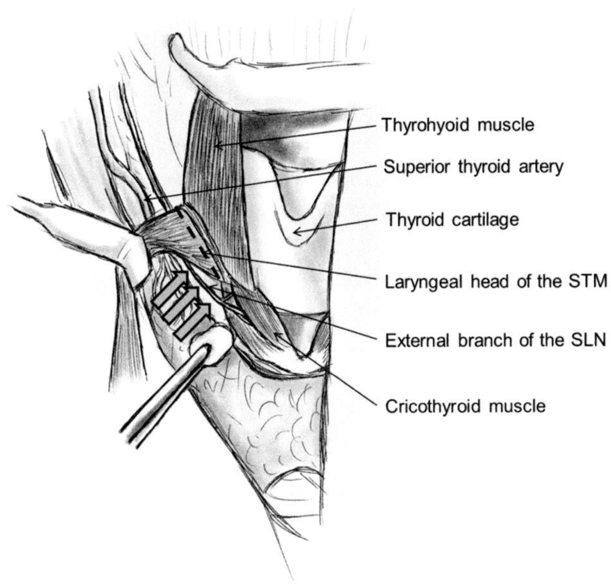


**Fig. 7.4** Stimulation of tissues parallel and underneath the laryngeal head of the sternothyroid muscle (marked with the dashed line) allows for the identification of the EBSLN in its distal course before entering the cricothyroid muscle. *STM* sternothyroid muscle, *SLN* superior laryngeal nerve (from Barczynski et al. [2]; with permission)

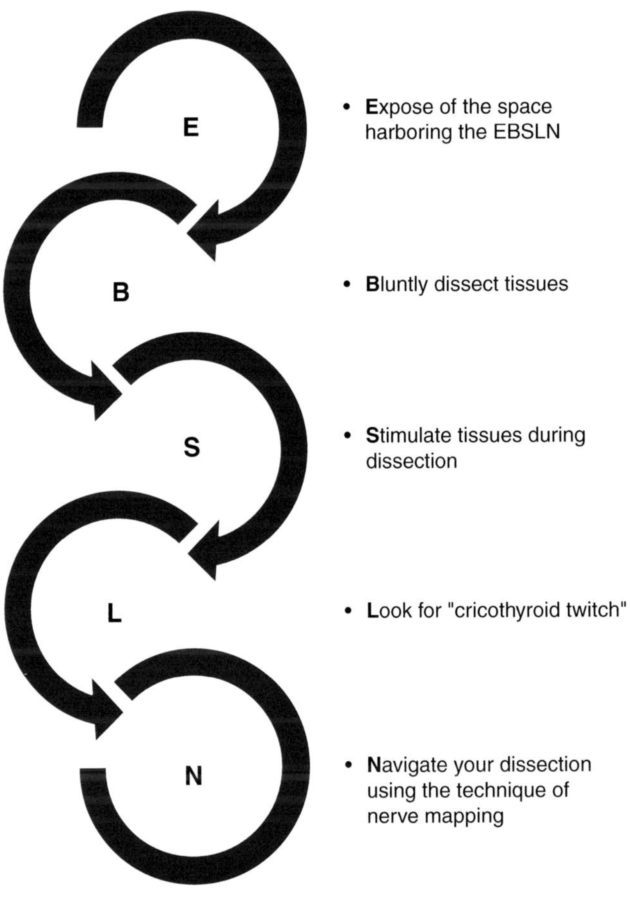


**Fig. 7.5** The mnemonic formula "EBSLN" summarizes surgical steps helpful in EBSLN identification with intraoperative nerve stimulation. *EBSLN* external branch of the superior laryngeal nerve

gland, in order to minimize the risk of inadvertent injury. Barczyński et al. [9] reported a randomized trial comparing 105 patients submitted to thyroidectomy identifying the EBSLN without any monitoring with 105 patients in whom EBSLN intraoperative monitoring was performed. The conclusion was that the nerve identification was less frequent in the first group (34.5%), compared to the second group (83.8%). In addition, there was a marked reduction of EBSLN injury in the second group, when compared to the first group (5% vs. 1%, respectively; $p = 0.02$).

Uludag et al. [10] also compared two groups of patients who underwent dissection of the superior thyroid pole: in Group 1, there was no attempt to identify the EBSLN, whereas in Group 2 intraoperative monitoring mapping of the EBSLN was undertaken. Nerve injury was documented in 8.6% of patients in Group 1, compared to 0.9% in Group 2 ($p = 0.015$).

Dionigi et al. [11] prospectively evaluated the frequency of injury of the EBSLN in 400 patients submitted to thyroidectomy in the three types of nerve according to Cernea's classification [1]. They found evidence of nerve injury of 4.9%, 11.2%, and 18.5%, respectively, among types 1, 2a, and 2b EBSLN ($p = 0.01$). They proposed the addition to routine evaluation of the EBSLN before and after the dissection of the superior thyroid pole (S1 and S2, respectively) to the algorithm already recommended by the International Neural Monitoring Study Group in 2011 [12].

Lee et al. [13] published a large series of patients submitted to thyroidectomy, divided into 2 Groups: in Group 1, they prospectively analyzed 490 thyroidectomies in which intraoperative monitoring of the EBSLN was employed; Group 2 included 500 operations without the use of intraoperative nerve monitoring, performed by the same surgeon. The use of nerve monitoring markedly improved the identification, especially among individuals with type 2b EBSLN.

Nayta et al. [14], in a recent meta-analysis, showed that injury of EBSLN occurs in up 58% of patients who underwent thyroidectomies, and the use of IONM resulted in a significant increase in EBSLN identification, decreasing the incidence of post-thyroidectomy voice disorders.

## Frequency of Use of EBSLN Intraoperative Nerve Monitoring

According to Barczyński et al. [15], the EBSLN intraoperative nerve monitoring during the dissection of the superior thyroid pole is more often employed by more experienced surgeons (61.4%), when compared with low-volume surgeons (15.8%), and this difference is significant ($p < 0.001$). This interesting finding supports the usefulness of intraoperative nerve monitoring of the EBSLN during thyroidectomy.

## Normative Features of EBSLN Intraoperative Monitoring

In 2013, Potenza et al. [16] presented normative features of EBSLN intraoperative monitoring and suggested that it may be used in order to facilitate the quantitative analysis of the physiologic status of the nerve during dissection of the superior thyroid pole. They performed a prospective non-randomized study of 72 patients submitted to thyroidectomy. All individuals underwent pre- and postoperative laryngoscopy, and those with abnormalities in the preoperative valuation were excluded. Initial intraoperative electrical stimulation in the region of the superior thyroid pole was done with 2 mA, in order to map the EBSLN, and was reduced to 1 mA after the nerve was identified. In all cases, the stimulation caused a CTM twitch. Conversely, a typical glottis waveform was observed in 78.1% of the EBSLN. The mean amplitude of the EBSLN complex was 269.9 (±178.6), compared with the mean RLN amplitude of 782.2 (±614.4) observed in the same side. As a matter of fact, there was no significant difference between the response of the EBSLN when stimulated with 1 mA (280.8 [±216.9] and those nerves stimulated with 2 mA (261.8 [±142.4] ($p$ = 0.7041). Regarding the results before and after the dissection of the superior thyroid pole, the mean amplitude of EMG response of the EBSLN obtained initially was 270.1 (±190.7), while the mean post-dissection response was 260.4 (±177.9). No significant difference was found between initial and final amplitudes of response ($p = 0.4689$).

In addition, in 2014, Darr et al. [17] reported, based on a prospective study undertaken in a cohort of 22 patients, that novel endotracheal tube (with an additional pair of superficial electrodes located on an anterior aspect of the tube) allows for quantifiable EBSLN EMG activity in 100% of cases. The clinical applicability of this observation is still under international and multi-institutional evaluation.

## Prognostic Parameters of the EBSLN and Change in Voice Quality Postoperatively

Iwata et al. reported recently on a prospective multicenter study which was conducted on patients undergoing thyroidectomies with intraoperative nerve monitoring. Electromyography waveforms of EBSLN stimulation before (S1) and after superior pole dissection (S2) were evaluated in this study using endotracheal tube (ETT) and cricothyroid intramuscular (CTM) electrodes. Voice outcomes were assessed using voice-related quality of life surveys and voice handicap index.

A total of 131 at-risk EBSLNs were evaluated in 80 patients. Two nerves showed loss of CTM twitch coupled with an absent S2 signal response. Complete EBSLN loss of signal was more likely with: (1) Cernea EBSLN anatomic classification Type 2B; (2) with a longer distance from the sternothyroid muscle insertion site; and (3) with larger lobar volumes ($P < 0.05$). Patients who experienced a more than 50% decrement in CTM amplitudes of S2 ($n = 7$) by CTM electrodes had a statistically significant decline in their voice outcomes compared to those who did not ($n = 69$) ($P < 0.05$). The authors concluded that patients experienced worse voice outcomes when at least one EBSLN response amplitude decreased by more than 50% after dissection when measured by CTM needle electrodes. CTM needle electrodes have an ability to measure finer amplitude changes compared to ETT electrodes, may represent a safe method to deduce subtle EBSLN injuries, and may serve to optimize voice outcomes during thyroidectomy. CTM needle electrodes are safe and tolerated well [18].

## Take-Home Messages

1. The EBSLN has a close anatomical relationship with the superior thyroid pedicle and is at risk of injury during dissection of these vessels in approximately one-third of patients (particularly in type 2b nerves).
2. The EBSLN injury is believed to be the most commonly underestimated morbidity following thyroid surgery.
3. Contrary to routine dissection of the recurrent laryngeal nerve, most surgeons tend to avoid rather than routinely expose and identify the EBSLN during thyroidectomy.
4. Thorough knowledge of the surgical anatomy of the EBSLN and its variations is mandatory to avoid damage to the nerve during thyroidectomy.
5. The laryngeal head of the sternothyroid muscle is a robust landmark for the course of the EBSLN as it descends along the inferior constrictor to the CTM.
6. CTM twitch and glottis EMG recordings are both methods of intraoperative neuromonitoring which are recommended in all cases of thyroid surgery which might jeopardize the EBSLN.
7. It is advisable to employ intraoperative monitoring not only of the inferior laryngeal nerve, but of the EBSLN as well, in order to facilitate its recognition and to reduce the risk of inadvertent injury, particularly when operating on female individuals and voice professionals.
8. A technique of togging the stimulator probe between the tissue of the superior thyroid pole vessels (with negative stimulation) and the region of the laryngeal head of the sternothyroid muscle (with positive stimulation) is recommended to assure preservation of the EBSLN.
9. Nerve stimulation can objectively identify the EBSLN, leading to a visible CTM twitch in all cases.
10. EMG activity can currently be quantified in nearly 80% of cases using standard EMG tubes, but in all patients using novel EMG tubes with anterior surface electrodes.

11. It is important to document the physiologic integrity of the nerve after the completion of the superior thyroid pole dissection; ideally, the obtained amplitude should be similar to the pre-dissection one.

## References


1. Cernea CR, Brandão LG, Hisham AN. Surgical anatomy of the superior laryngeal nerve. In: Randolph GW, editor. Surgery of thyroid and parathyroid gland. Philadelphia: Elsevier Saunders; 2018. p. 316–25.
2. Barczyński M, Randolph GW, Cernea CR, et al. External branch of the superior laryngeal nerve monitoring during thyroid and parathyroid surgery: International Neural Monitoring Study Group standard guidelines. Laryngoscope. 2013;123(suppl 4):S1–S14.
3. Wang K, Cai H, Kong D, et al. The identification, preservation, and classification of the external branch of the superior laryngeal nerve in thyroidectomy. World J Surg. 2017;41:2521–9. https://doi.org/10.1007/s00268-017-4046-z.
4. Cernea CR, Ferraz AR, Nishio S, et al. Surgical anatomy of the external branch of the superior laryngeal nerve. Head Neck. 1992;14:380–3. https://doi.org/10.1002/hed.2880140507.
5. Cernea CR, Ferraz AR, Furlani J, et al. Identification of the external branch of the superior laryngeal nerve during thyroidectomy. Am J Surg. 1992;164:634–9. https://doi.org/10.1016/s0002-9610(05)80723-8.
6. Furlan JC, Cordeiro AC, Brandão LG. Study of some "intrinsic risk factors" that can enhance an iatrogenic injury of the external branch of the superior laryngeal nerve. Otolaryngol Head Neck Surg. 2003;128(3):396–400.
7. Moosman DA, DeWeese MS. The external laryngeal nerve as related to thyroidectomy. Surg Gynecol Obstet. 1968;129:1011–6.
8. Teitelbaum WBL. Superior laryngeal nerve injury from thyroid surgery. Head Neck. 1995;17:36–40.
9. Barczyński M, Konturek A, Stopa M, Honowska A, Nowak W. Randomized controlled trial of visualization versus neuromonitoring of the external branch of the superior laryngeal nerve during thyroidectomy. World J Surg. 2012;36(6):1340–7.
10. Uludag M, Aygun N, Kartal K, et al. Contribution of intraoperative neural monitoring to preservation of the external branch of the superior laryngeal nerve: a randomized prospective clinical trial. Langenbeck's Arch Surg. 2017;402(6):965–76.
11. Dionigi G, Kim HY, Randolph GW, et al. Prospective validation study of Cernea classification for predicting EMG alterations of the external branch of the superior laryngeal nerve. Surg Today. 2016;46(7):785–91.
12. Randolph GW, et al. Electrophysiologic recurrent laryngeal nerve monitoring during thyroid and parathyroid surgery: international standards guideline statement. Laryngoscope. 2011;121(Suppl 1):1–16.
13. Lee J, Fraser S, Glover A, Sidhu S. Prospective evaluation of the utility of routine neuromonitoring for an established thyroid surgical practice. ANZ J Surg. 2017;87(10):E138–42.
14. Naytah M, Ibrahim I, da Silva S. Importance of incorporating intraoperative neuromonitoring of the external branch of the superior laryngeal nerve in thyroidectomy: a review and meta-analysis study. Head Neck. 2019;41(6):2034–41. https://doi.org/10.1002/hed.25669. Epub 2019 Feb 1.
15. Barczyński M, Randolph GW, Cernea C, International Neural Monitoring Study Group in Thyroid and Parathyroid Surgery. International survey on the identification and neural monitoring of the EBSLN during thyroidectomy. Laryngoscope. 2016;126(1):285–91.
16. Andre S, Potenza A, Phelan EA, Claudio R, Cernea CR, et al. Normative intra-operative electrophysiologic waveform analysis of superior laryngeal nerve external branch and recurrent laryngeal nerve in patients undergoing thyroid surgery. World J Surg. 2013;37:2336–42.
17. Darr EA, Tufano RP, Ozdemir S, Kamani D, Hurwitz S, Randolph G. Superior laryngeal nerve quantitative intraoperative monitoring is possible in all thyroid surgeries. Laryngoscope. 2014;124(4):1035–41.
18. Iwata AJ, Liddy W, Barczyński M, Wu CW, Huang TY, Van Slycke S, et al. Superior laryngeal nerve signal attenuation influences voice outcomes in thyroid surgery. Laryngoscope. 2021;131(6):1436–42.

# 8 Intraoperative Neurophysiologic Monitoring for the Recurrent Laryngeal Nerve: Case Illustrations

Joseph DiAngelo, Pedro Garcia, Thomas Lopazanski, Alan D. Deutsch, and Alexander L. Shifrin

The following illustrations were obtained during intraoperative neurophysiologic monitoring of the recurrent laryngeal nerve (RLN). Recording electrodes are incorporated into an endotracheal tube (ETT) (Nuvasive® EMG Endotracheal Tube; San Diego, CA), where after intubation by the anesthesiologist, the electrodes lie at the level of the vocal cords. Flexible laryngoscopy can be performed after intubation to ensure adequate electrode alignment with the vocal cords. Stimulation is conducted with the use of a Prass standard monopolar cathode stimulator (Medtronic Xomed Inc.®; Minneapolis, MN). A reference anode needle electrode is placed in the trapezius muscle. Stimulus intensities of 0.5–4 milliamps (mA) are utilized. The surgeon is handed the sterile probe after exposure and the surgeon can then stimulate neural and non-neural structures throughout the course of surgery. When stimulating the RLN directly, a triggered action potential waveform is generated and the surgeon is notified of a positive response. When stimulation is not over the RLN, no response is generated and the surgeon is notified of the absence of a triggered waveform. Audio on the recording equipment allows the surgeon to hear a positive response in real time. In between direct stimulation, free running EMG activity is monitored throughout the surgical procedure from the recording electrodes in the ETT. All waveforms and data were obtained utilizing Cadwell Cascade® (Kennewick, WA) intraoperative monitoring recording equipment (Figs. 8.1, 8.2, and 8.3).

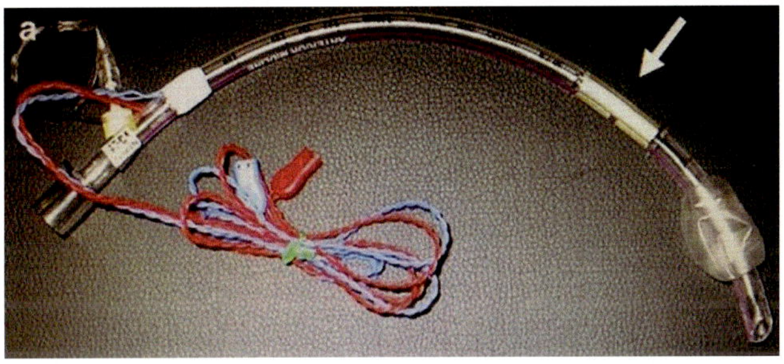


**Fig. 8.1** Nuvasive® EMG endotracheal tube. *Arrow* indicates the recoding electrodes


J. DiAngelo · P. Garcia · T. Lopazanski · A. D. Deutsch
Monmouth Ocean Neurology, Neptune, NJ, USA

A. L. Shifrin (✉)
Surgical Director of Endocrinology, Atlantic Health CentraState Medical Center, Freehold, NJ, USA



A. L. Shifrin et al. (eds.), *Atlas of Intraoperative Cranial Nerve Monitoring in Thyroid and Head and Neck Surgery*,
https://doi.org/10.1007/978-3-031-24613-5_8

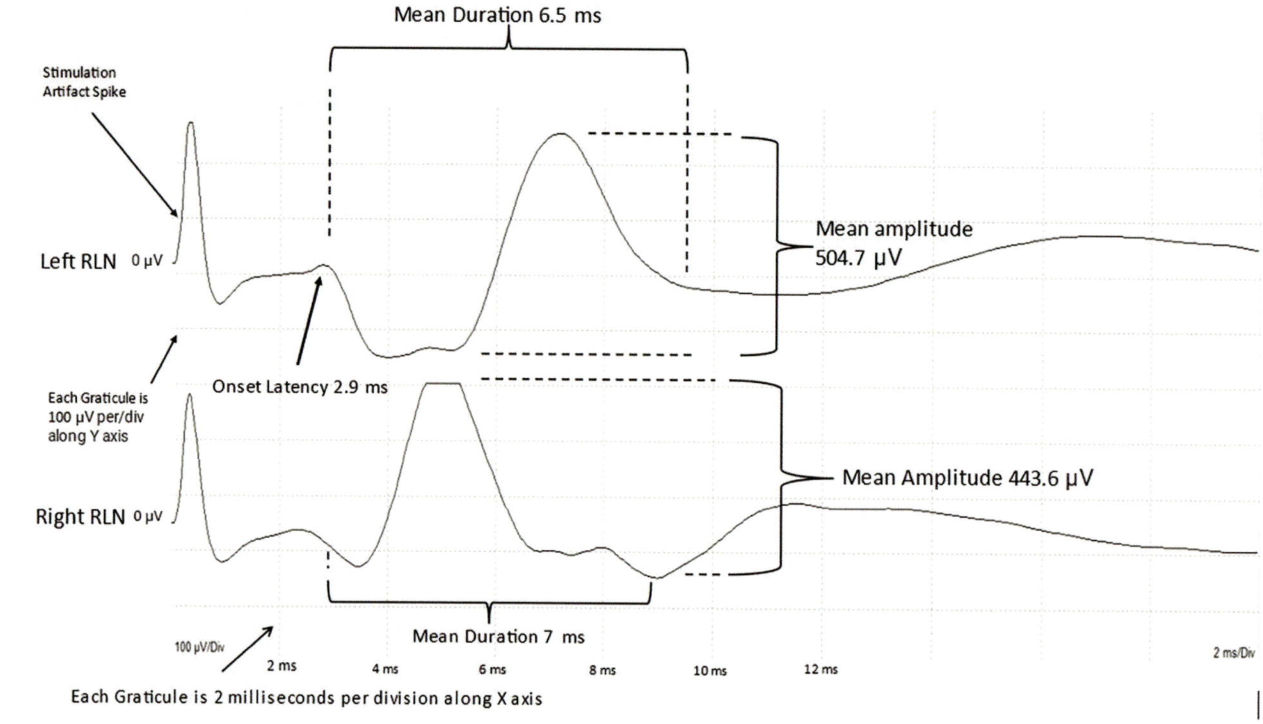


**Fig. 8.2** A triggered action potential derived from direct stimulation of the left and right RLN at a stimulus intensity of 1.5 mA

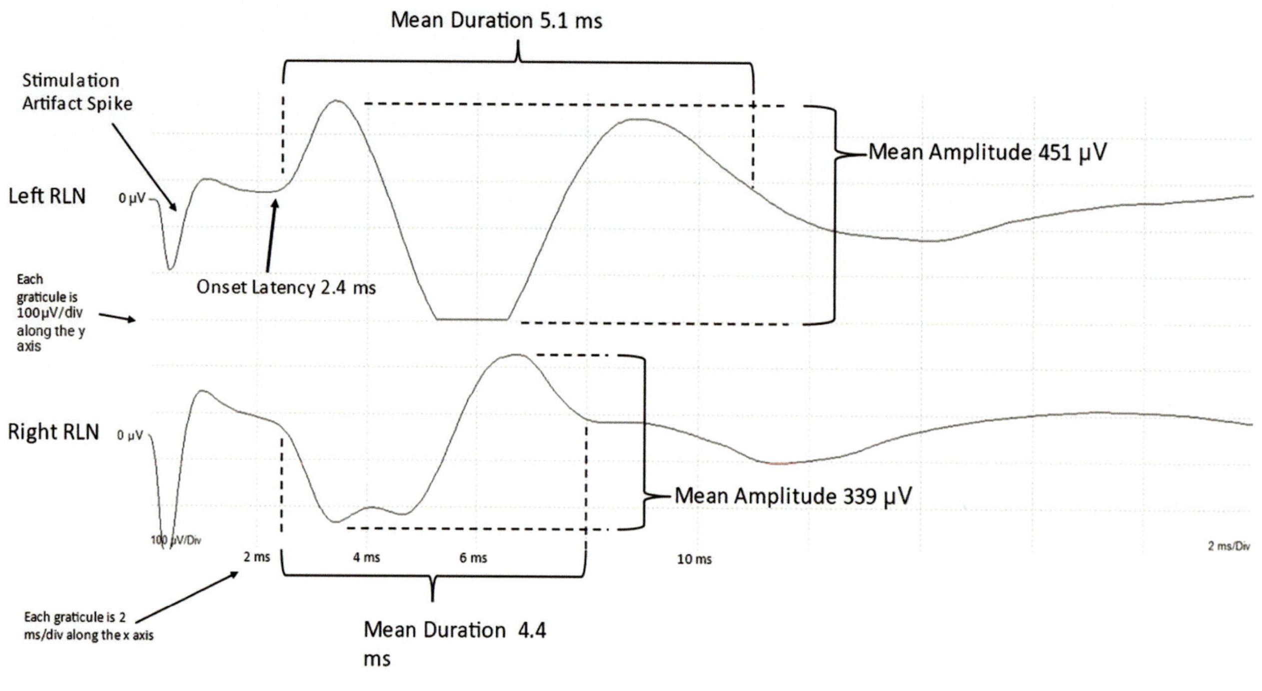


**Fig. 8.3** A triggered action potential derived from direct stimulation of the left and right RLN at a stimulus intensity of 2.0 mA

## Further Reading

Cirocchi R, Arezzo A, D'Andrea V, Abraha I, Popivanov GI, Avenia N, et al. Intraoperative neuromonitoring versus visual nerve identification for prevention of recurrent laryngeal nerve injury in adults undergoing thyroid surgery. Cochrane Database Syst Rev. 2019;1(1):CD01248.

Liddy W, Lawson BR, Barber SR, Kamani D, Shama M, Soylu S, et al. Anterior laryngeal electrodes for recurrent laryngeal nerve monitoring during thyroid and parathyroid surgery: new expanded options for neural monitoring. Laryngoscope. 2018;128(12):2910–5. https://doi.org/10.1002/lary.27362. Epub 2018 Nov 12.

Randolph GW. The recurrent and superior laryngeal nerves. New York: Springer; 2016.

Randolph GW, Dralle H, International Intraoperative Monitoring Study Group, et al. Electrophysiologic recurrent laryngeal nerve monitoring during thyroid and parathyroid surgery: international standards guideline statement. Laryngoscope. 2011;121(Suppl):S1–16. https://doi.org/10.1002/lary.21119.

Randolph GW, Kamani D. Intraoperative electrophysiologic monitoring of the recurrent laryngeal nerve during thyroid and parathyroid surgery: experience with 1,381 nerves at risk. Laryngoscope. 2017;127(1):280–6.

Romano N, Federici M, Castaldi A. Imaging of cranial nerves: a pictorial overview. Insights Imaging. 2019;10:33.

Rustad WH. The recurrent laryngeal nerves in thyroid surgery. New York: Thomas; 1956.

Wu CW, Huang TY, Randolph GW, Barczyński M, Schneider R, Chiang FY, et al. Informed consent for intraoperative neural monitoring in thyroid and parathyroid surgery—consensus statement of the International Neural Monitoring Study Group. Front Endocrinol. 2021;12:795281. https://doi.org/10.3389/fendo.2021.795281.

# 9 Intraoperative Neurophysiological Monitoring for the External Branch of the Superior Laryngeal Nerve: Case Illustrations

Joseph DiAngelo, Pedro Garcia, Thomas Lopazanski, Alan D. Deutsch, and Alexander L. Shifrin

The superior laryngeal nerve is a branch of the vagus nerve (CN X) and divides into the internal and external branches of the superior laryngeal nerve. The external branch of the superior laryngeal nerve (EBSLN) supplies motor enervation to the cricothyroid muscle. During thyroid surgery the EBSLN can be monitored by placing paired subdermal needle electrodes into the cricothyroid muscle (Fig. 9.1). An endotracheal tube (ETT) incorporating electrodes which lie at the level of the vocal cords after intubation can also be utilized for monitoring of the EBSLN. Utilizing recording intraoperative monitoring equipment, free running EMG activity from the cricothyroid muscle and the ETT can be monitored for any indirect activation of the EBSLN. Direct stimulation of the EBSLN can also be performed with the use of a Prass monopolar cathode stimulator (Medtronic Xomed Inc.®; Minneapolis, MN) with a reference anode electrode placed in the trapezius muscle. Stimulation intensities of 0.5–4 milliamps (mA) are used. All waveforms and data were obtained utilizing Cadwell Cascade® (Kennewick, WA) intraoperative monitoring recording equipment (Figs. 9.2 and 9.3).

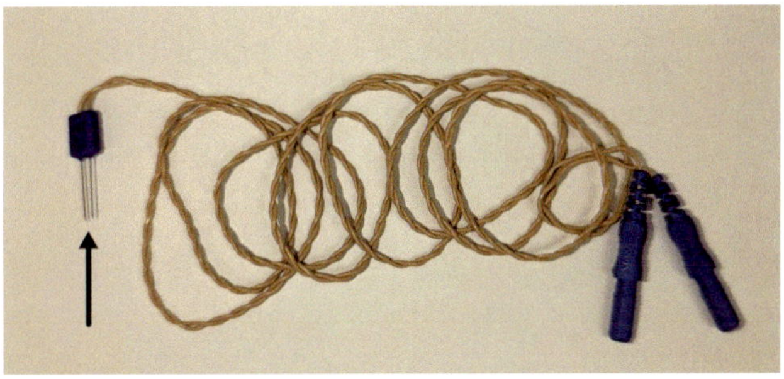

**Fig. 9.1** Paired subdermal needle electrodes (Medtronic Xomed, Inc.®) placed into the cricothyroid muscle for monitoring of the EBSLN. The arrow points to the paired needle portion of the electrodes used for recording

J. DiAngelo · P. Garcia · T. Lopazanski · A. D. Deutsch
Monmouth Ocean Neurology, Neptune, NJ, USA

A. L. Shifrin (✉)
Surgical Director of Endocrinology, Atlantic Health CentraState Medical Center, Freehold, NJ, USA


A. L. Shifrin et al. (eds.), *Atlas of Intraoperative Cranial Nerve Monitoring in Thyroid and Head and Neck Surgery*,
https://doi.org/10.1007/978-3-031-24613-5_9

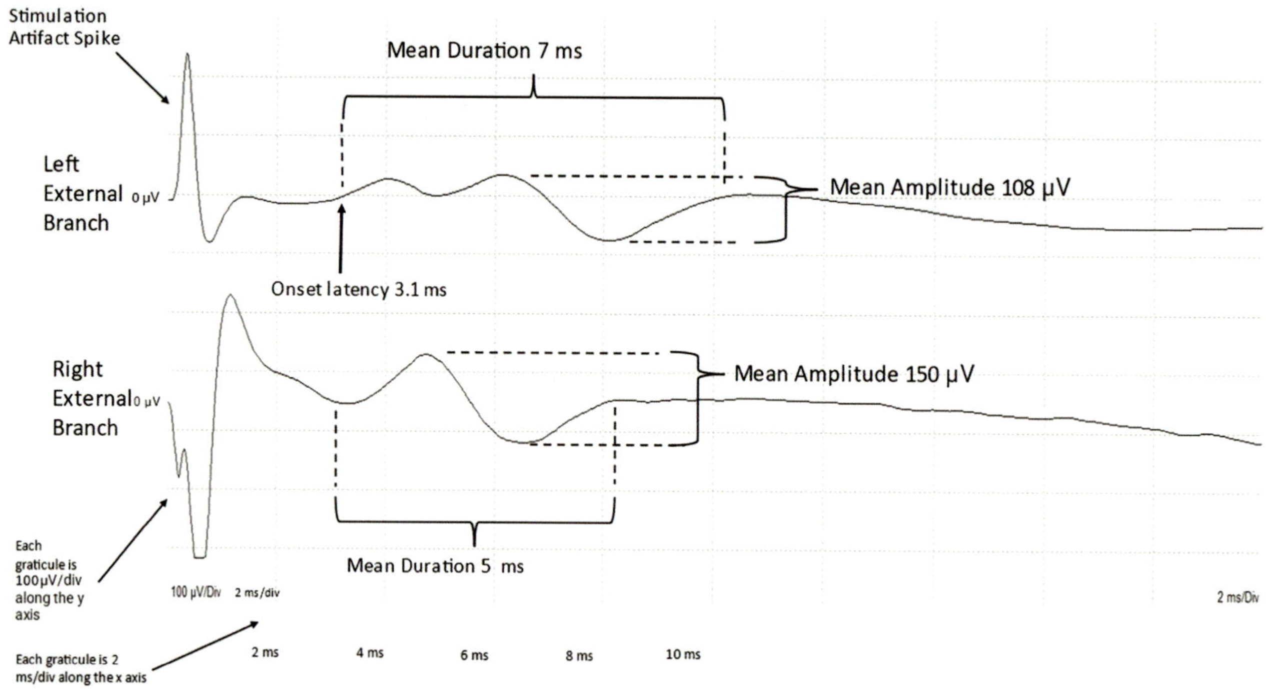


**Fig. 9.2** Direct stimulation of the left and right EBSLN (labeled External Branch) at a stimulus intensity of 2.0 mA recording from ETT-placed electrodes

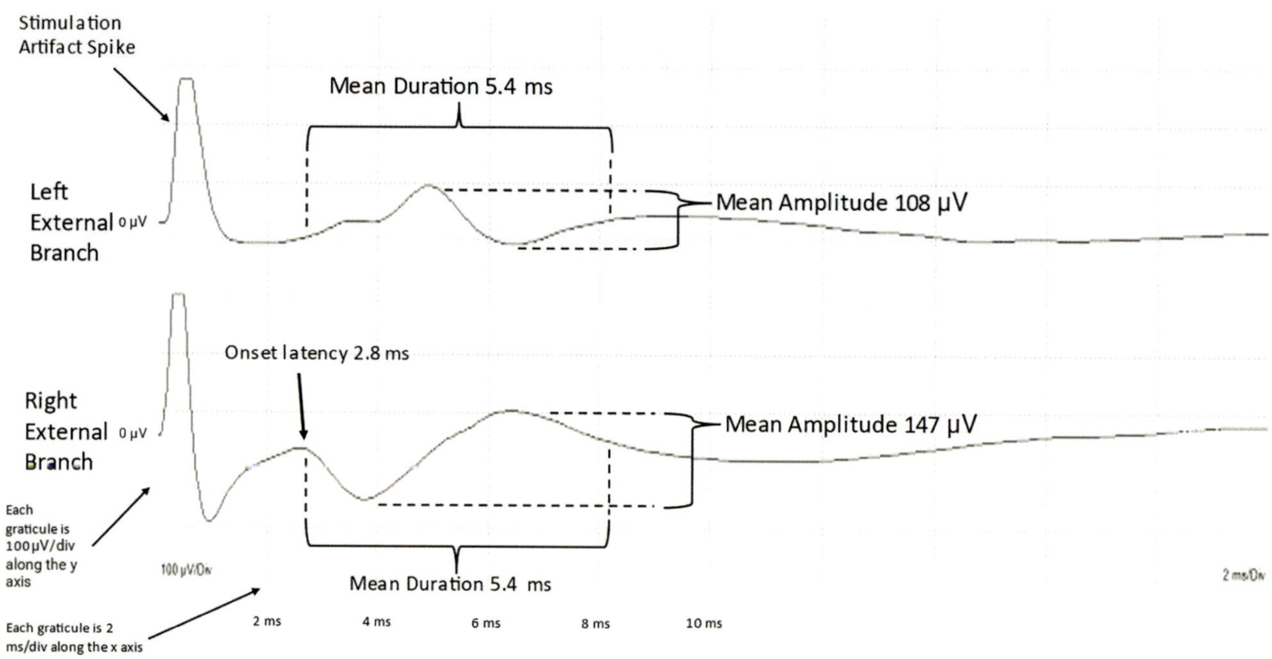


**Fig. 9.3** Direct stimulation of the left and right EBSLN (labeled External Branch) at a stimulus intensity of 2.5 mA recording from cricothyroid-placed electrodes

## Further Reading

Cernea CR, Ferraz AR, Nishio S, Dutra A Jr, Hojaij FC, Dos Santos LRM. Surgical anatomy of the external branch of the superior laryngeal nerve. Head Neck. 1992;14:380–3. https://doi.org/10.1002/hed.2880140507.

Cirocchi R, Arezzo A, D'Andrea V, Abraha I, Popivanov GI, Avenia N, Gerardi C, et al. Intraoperative neuromonitoring versus visual nerve identification for prevention of recurrent laryngeal nerve injury in adults undergoing thyroid surgery. Cochrane Database Syst Rev. 2019;1(1):CD012483. https://doi.org/10.1002/14651858.CD012483.pub2.

Iwata AJ, Liddy W, Barczyński M, Wu CW, Huang TY, Van Slycke S, Schneider R, Dionigi G, Dralle H, Cernea CR, Kamani D, Ahmed AH, Okose OC, Wang B, Randolph GW. Superior laryngeal nerve signal attenuation influences voice outcomes in thyroid surgery. Laryngoscope. 2021;131(6):1436–42. https://doi.org/10.1002/lary.29413.

Randolph GW. The recurrent and superior laryngeal nerves. New York: Springer; 2016.

Randolph GW, Dralle H, et al. Electrophysiologic recurrent laryngeal nerve monitoring during thyroid and parathyroid surgery: international standards guideline statement. Laryngoscope. 2011;121(Suppl):1–16. https://doi.org/10.1002/lary.21119.

Randolph GW, Kamani D. Intraoperative electrophysiologic monitoring of the recurrent laryngeal nerve during thyroid and parathyroid surgery: experience with 1,381 nerves at risk. Laryngoscope. 2017;127(1):280–6.

Romano N, Federici M, Castaldi A. Imaging of cranial nerves: a pictorial overview. Insights Imaging. 2019;10:33.

Rustad WH. The recurrent laryngeal nerves in thyroid surgery. New York: Thomas; 1956.

Sakorafas GH, Kokoropoulos P, Lappas C, Sampanis D, Smyrniotis V. External branch of the superior laryngeal nerve: applied surgical anatomy and implications in thyroid surgery. Am Surg. 2012;78(9):986–91. PMID: 22964209.

Sañudo JR, Maranillo E, León X, Mirapeix RM, Orús C, Quer M. An anatomical study of anastomoses between the laryngeal nerves. Laryngoscope. 1999;109(6):983–7. https://doi.org/10.1097/00005537-199906000-00026. PMID: 10369294.

Wu CW, Huang TY, Randolph GW, Barczyński M, Schneider R, Chiang FY, et al. Informed consent for intraoperative neural monitoring in thyroid and parathyroid surgery—consensus statement of the International Neural Monitoring Study Group. Front Endocrinol. 2021;12:795281. https://doi.org/10.3389/fendo.2021.795281.

Wu CW, Randolph GW, Barczyński M, Schneider R, Chiang FY, Huang TY, et al. Training courses in laryngeal nerve monitoring in thyroid and parathyroid surgery. The INMSG consensus statement. Front Endocrinol. 2021;12:705346. https://doi.org/10.3389/fendo.2021.705346.

# Intraoperative Neurophysiological Monitoring for the Vagus Nerve: Case Illustrations

10

Joseph DiAngelo, Pedro Garcia, Thomas Lopazanski, Alan D. Deutsch, and Alexander L. Shifrin

The vagus nerve, cranial nerve 10 (CN X), runs from the medulla into the neck. The relevant bilateral branches of the nerve pertinent to this atlas include the recurrent laryngeal nerve and the superior laryngeal nerve, which further branches into internal and external branches. There is a potential risk for injury to the vagus nerve during head and neck surgeries. The vagus nerve can be monitored by use of an endotracheal tube containing recording electrodes which after intubation lie at the level of the vocal cords for recording the distal recurrent laryngeal nerve (RLN). Needle electrodes are also placed into the cricothyroid muscle for monitoring of the external branch of the superior laryngeal nerve (EBSLN). Please see Chaps. 8 and 9 for monitoring techniques for the RLN and EBSLN. The vagus nerve is directly stimulated by the surgeon in the neck with the use of a Prass monopolar cathode stimulator (Medtronic Xomed Inc.®; Minneapolis, MN) and reference anode needle electrode placed into the ipsilateral trapezius muscle. Stimulus intensities of 0.5–2 milliamps (mA) are most frequently used. Free running EMG for any indirect stimulation of the vagus nerve recording from the above electrodes in the ETT and cricothyroid muscle is also monitored. All waveforms and data were obtained utilizing Cadwell Cascade® (Kennewick, WA) intraoperative monitoring recording equipment (Figs. 10.1 and 10.2).

J. DiAngelo · P. Garcia · T. Lopazanski · A. D. Deutsch
Monmouth Ocean Neurology, Neptune, NJ, USA

A. L. Shifrin (✉)
Surgical Director of Endocrinology, Atlantic Health CentraState Medical Center, Freehold, NJ, USA


A. L. Shifrin et al. (eds.), *Atlas of Intraoperative Cranial Nerve Monitoring in Thyroid and Head and Neck Surgery*,
https://doi.org/10.1007/978-3-031-24613-5_10

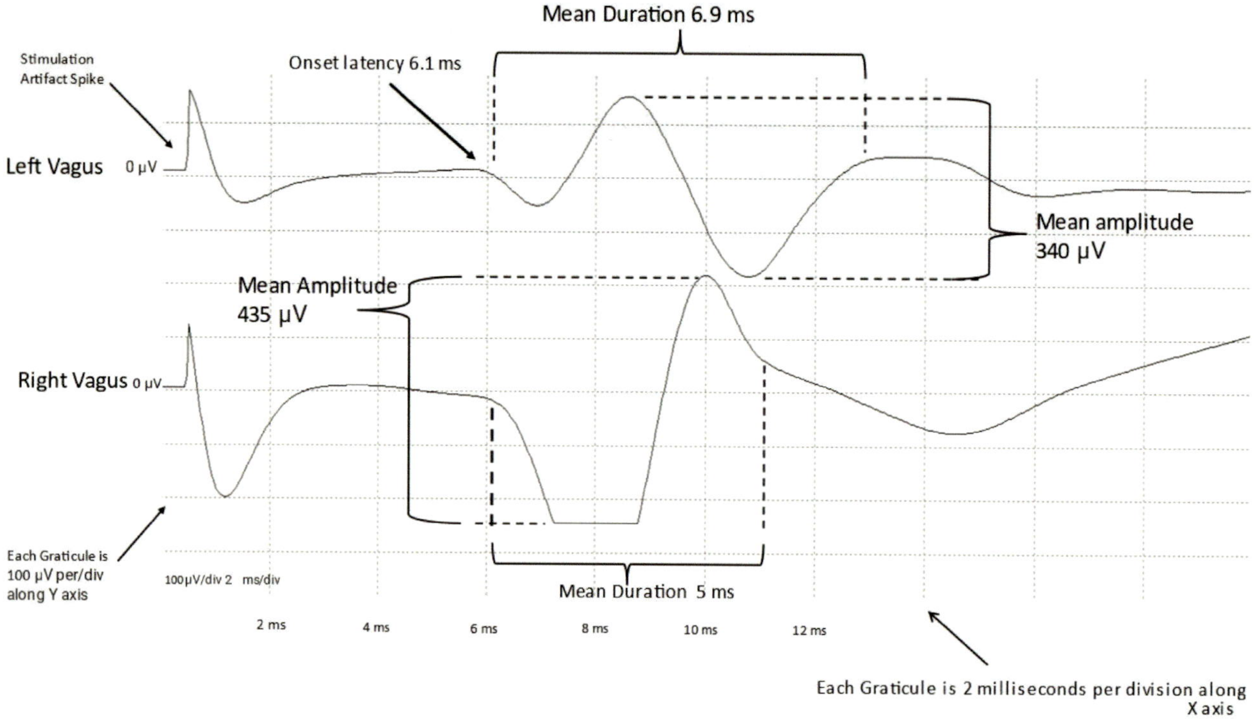


**Fig. 10.1** Triggered waveforms by direct stimulation of the left and right vagus nerve in the neck at a stimulation intensity of 2.0 mA. Note the delay in the onset latency as compared to stimulation of the RLN and EBSLN (*see* Chaps. 8 and 9), given the longer course and stimulation of the vagus nerves more proximally in the neck

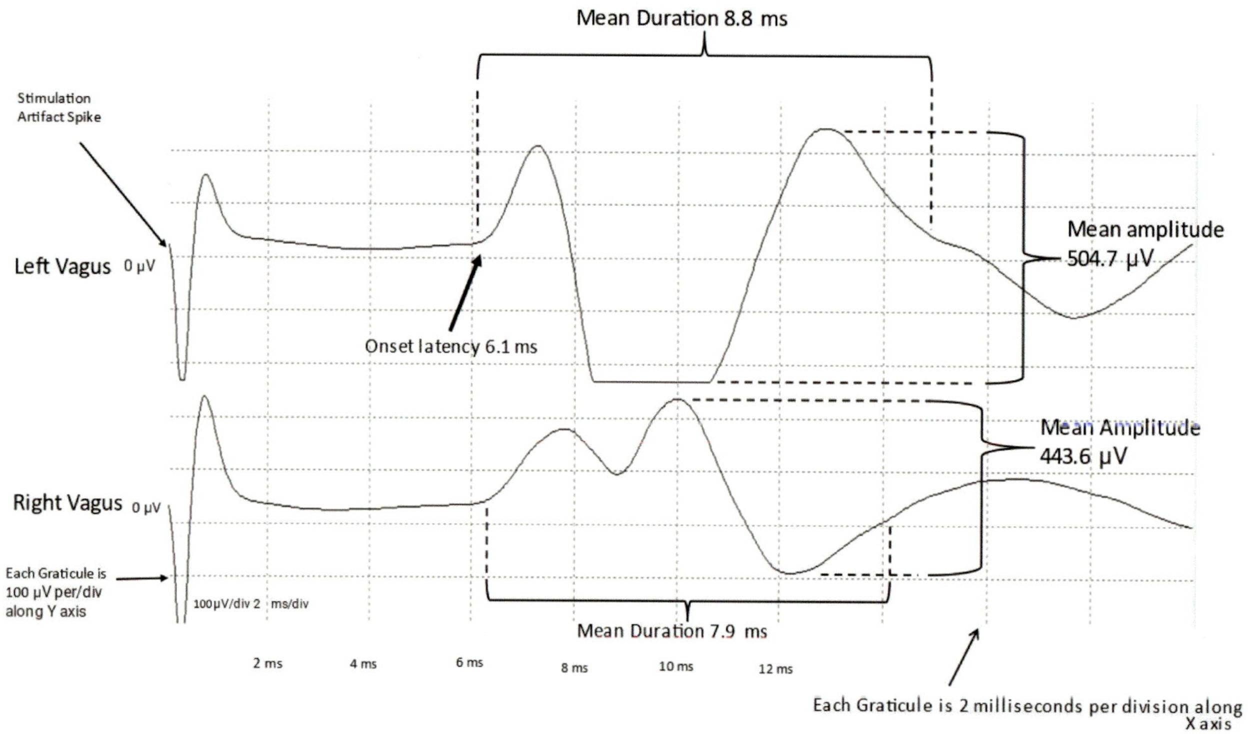


**Fig. 10.2** Triggered waveforms by direct stimulation of the left and right vagus nerve in the neck at a stimulus intensity of 2.0 mA. Note the delay in the onset latency as compared to stimulation of the RLN and EBSLN (*see* Chaps. 8 and 9), given the longer course and stimulation of the vagus nerves more proximally in the neck

## Further Reading

Cirocchi R, Arezzo A, D'Andrea V, Abraha I, Popivanov GI, Avenia N, et al. Intraoperative neuromonitoring versus visual nerve identification for prevention of recurrent laryngeal nerve injury in adults undergoing thyroid surgery. Cochrane Database Syst Rev. 2019;1(1):CD012483. https://doi.org/10.1002/14651858.CD012483.pub2.

Deniwar A, Kandil E, Randolph G. Electrophysiological neural monitoring of the laryngeal nerves in thyroid surgery: review of the current literature. Gland Surg. 2015;4(5):368–75.

Liddy W, Barber S, Cinquepalmi M, Lin BM, Patricio S, Kyriazidis N, et al. The electrophysiology of thyroid surgery: electrophysiologic and muscular responses with stimulation of the vagus nerve, recurrent laryngeal nerve, and external branch of the superior laryngeal nerve. Laryngoscope. 2017;127(3):764–71. https://doi.org/10.1002/lary.26147. Epub 2016 Jul 4.

Orloff LA. Noninvasive continuous vagal-nerve monitoring, harnessing the primitive laryngeal adductor reflex, is on the horizon. Clin Thyroidol. 2019;31:490–2.

Randolph GW, Dralle H, et al. Electrophysiologic recurrent laryngeal nerve monitoring during thyroid and parathyroid surgery: international standards guideline statement. Laryngoscope. 2011;121(Suppl):1–16. https://doi.org/10.1002/lary.21119.

Voskanian IE, Kolomeĭtsev SN, Shniukov RV. Risk factors and prevention of injuries to the cranial nerves in reconstructive surgery of the carotid arteries. Angiol Sosud Khir. 2005;11(2):96–103.

Wu CW, Huang TY, Randolph GW, Barczyński M, Schneider R, Chiang FY, et al. Informed consent for intraoperative neural monitoring in thyroid and parathyroid surgery—consensus statement of the International Neural Monitoring Study Group. Front Endocrinol. 2021;12:795281. https://doi.org/10.3389/fendo.2021.795281.

Wu CW, Randolph GW, Barczyński M, Schneider R, Chiang FY, Huang TY, et al. Training courses in laryngeal nerve monitoring in thyroid and parathyroid surgery. The INMSG consensus statement. Front Endocrinol. 2021;12:705346. https://doi.org/10.3389/fendo.2021.705346.

# Intraoperative Neurophysiological Monitoring for the Spinal Accessory Nerve: Case Illustrations

11

Joseph DiAngelo, Pedro Garcia, Thomas Lopazanski, Alan D. Deutsch, and Alexander L. Shifrin

The spinal accessory nerve, cranial nerve XI, begins at the level of the medulla and travels through the neck to supply motor innervation to the trapezius and sternocleidomastoid (SCM) muscles. The spinal accessory nerve has the potential for injury during radical head and neck surgeries resulting in weakness of the muscles supplied. Intraoperative neurophysiologic monitoring is performed by placing dual subdermal needle electrodes into the ipsilateral upper trapezius muscle on the side of dissection. A Prass probe monopolar cathode stimulator (Medtronic Xomed Inc.®; Minneapolis, MN) with an adjacent anode reference needle electrode placed in nearby muscle is used by the surgeon to directly stimulate when the spinal accessory nerve is localized. Stimulus intensities of 0.5–4 milliamps (mA) are utilized. Free running EMG activity is also monitored from the trapezius muscle electrodes during the course of surgery for any indirect stimulation of the spinal accessory nerve. All waveforms and data were obtained utilizing Cadwell Cascade® (Kennewick, MN) intraoperative monitoring recording equipment (Figs. 11.1 and 11.2).

J. DiAngelo · P. Garcia · T. Lopazanski · A. D. Deutsch
Monmouth Ocean Neurology, Neptune, NJ, USA

A. L. Shifrin (✉)
Surgical Director of Endocrinology, Atlantic Health CentraState Medical Center, Freehold, NJ, USA


A. L. Shifrin et al. (eds.), *Atlas of Intraoperative Cranial Nerve Monitoring in Thyroid and Head and Neck Surgery*,
https://doi.org/10.1007/978-3-031-24613-5_11

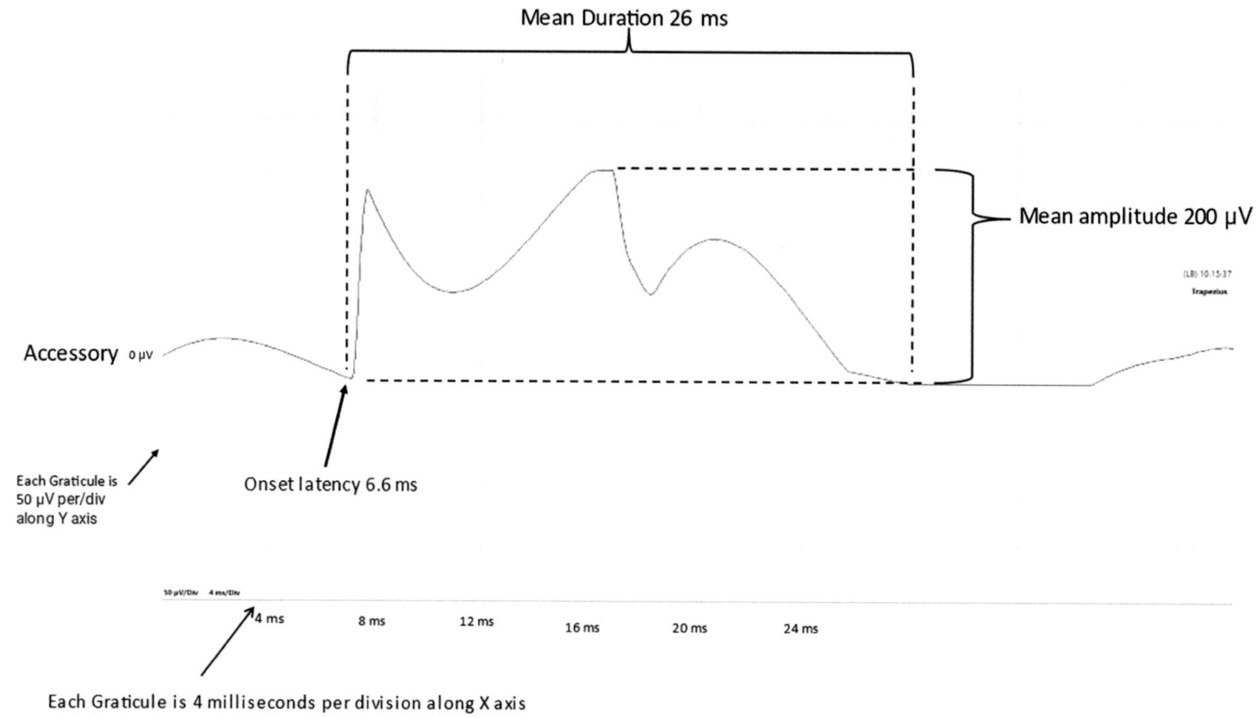


**Fig. 11.1** Direct stimulation of the spinal accessory nerve in the neck at a stimulus intensity of 2.0 mA and recording from the ipsilateral trapezius muscle electrodes

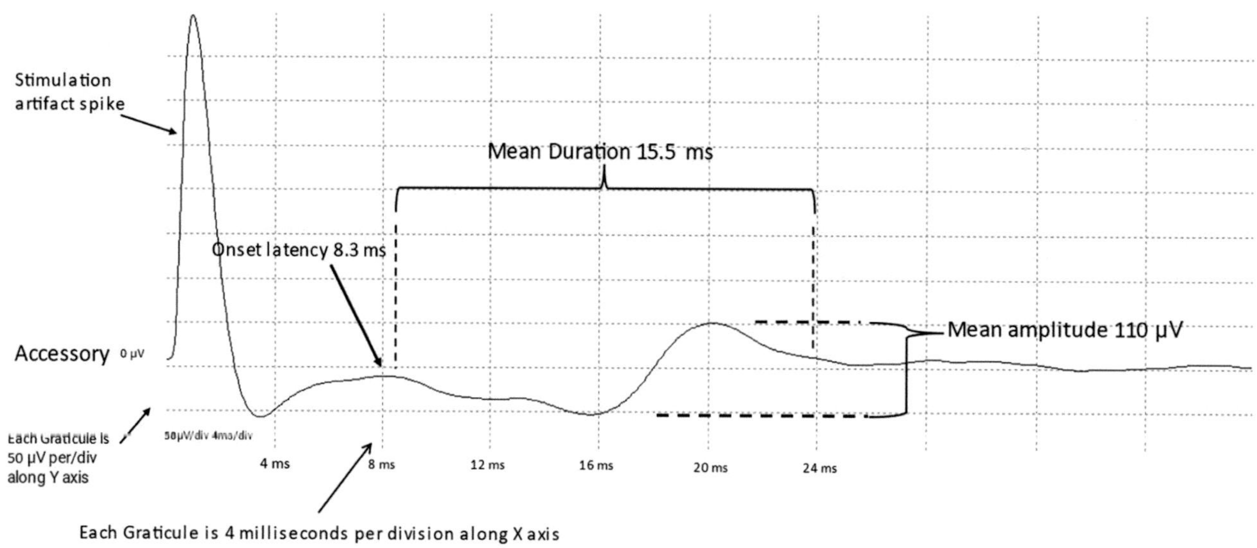


**Fig. 11.2** Direct stimulation of the spinal accessory nerve at a stimulus intensity of 1.5 mA while recording from the ipsilateral trapezius muscle electrodes

## Further Reading

Lanisnik B, Zargi M, Rodi Z. Identification of three anatomical patterns of the spinal accessory nerve in the neck by neurophysiological mapping. Radiol Oncol. 2014;48(4):387–92.

Lee CH, Huang NC, Chen HC, Chen MK. Minimizing shoulder syndrome with intra-operative spinal accessory nerve monitoring for neck dissection. Acta Otorhinolaryngol Ital. 2013;33(2):93–6.

Morris LGT, Ziff DJS, DeLacure MD. Malpractice litigation after surgical injury of the spinal accessory nerve: an evidence-based analysis. Arch Otolaryngol Head Neck Surg. 2008;134(1):102–7.

Popovski V, Benedetti A, Popovic-Monevska D, Grcev A, Stamatoski A, Zhivadinovik J. Spinal accessory nerve preservation in modified neck dissections: surgical and functional outcomes. Acta Otorhinolaryngol Ital. 2017;37(5):368–74.

Skinner SA. Neurophysiologic monitoring of the spinal accessory nerve, hypoglossal nerve and the spinomedullary region. J Clin Neurophysiol. 2011;11(6):587–98.

Wiater JM, Bigliani LU. Spinal accessory nerve injury. Clin Orthop Relat Res. 1999;368:5–16.

# 12 Intraoperative Neurophysiological Monitoring for the Hypoglossal Nerve: Case Illustrations

Joseph DiAngelo, Pedro Garcia, Thomas Lopazanski, Alan D. Deutsch, and Alexander L. Shifrin

The hypoglossal nerve, cranial nerve XII, arises from the medulla traveling out of the skull through the hypoglossal canal into the neck and submandibular area to supply motor innervation to all the muscles of the tongue. The hypoglossal nerve has the potential to be injured during radical head and neck surgeries. The hypoglossal nerve can be monitored intraoperatively by placing dual subdermal needle electrodes into the genioglossus muscle. Indirect monitoring of the hypoglossal nerve can be performed by free running EMG activity from the genioglossus muscle electrodes. Triggered direct stimulation of the hypoglossal nerve when localized is performed by the surgeon using a Prass monopolar cathode stimulator (Medtronic Xomed Inc.®; Minneapolis, MN) at stimulation intensities ranging from 0.5 to 4.0 milliamps (mA). All waveforms and data were obtained utilizing Cadwell Cascade® (Kennewick, WA) intraoperative monitoring recording equipment (Figs. 12.1 and 12.2).

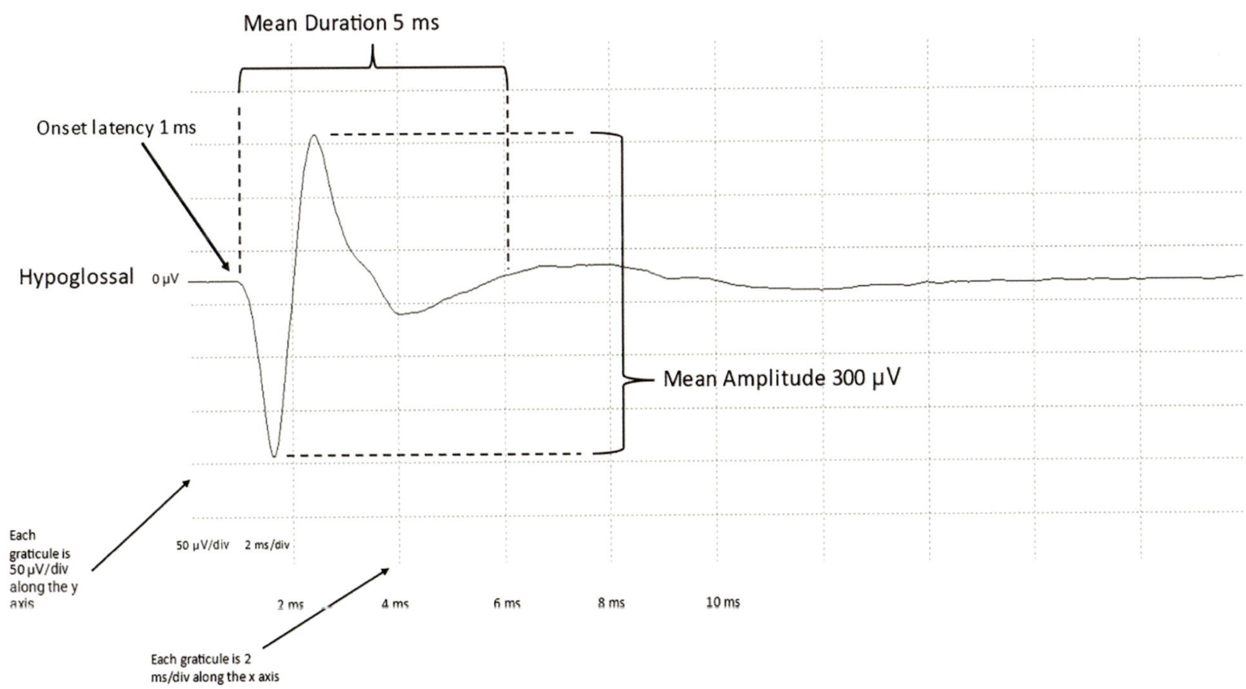


**Fig. 12.1** Direct stimulation of the hypoglossal nerve recording from the genioglossus muscle at a stimulation intensity of 1.5 mA

J. DiAngelo · P. Garcia · T. Lopazanski · A. D. Deutsch
Monmouth Ocean Neurology, Neptune, NJ, USA

A. L. Shifrin (✉)
Surgical Director of Endocrinology, Atlantic Health CentraState Medical Center, Freehold, NJ, USA


A. L. Shifrin et al. (eds.), *Atlas of Intraoperative Cranial Nerve Monitoring in Thyroid and Head and Neck Surgery*,
https://doi.org/10.1007/978-3-031-24613-5_12

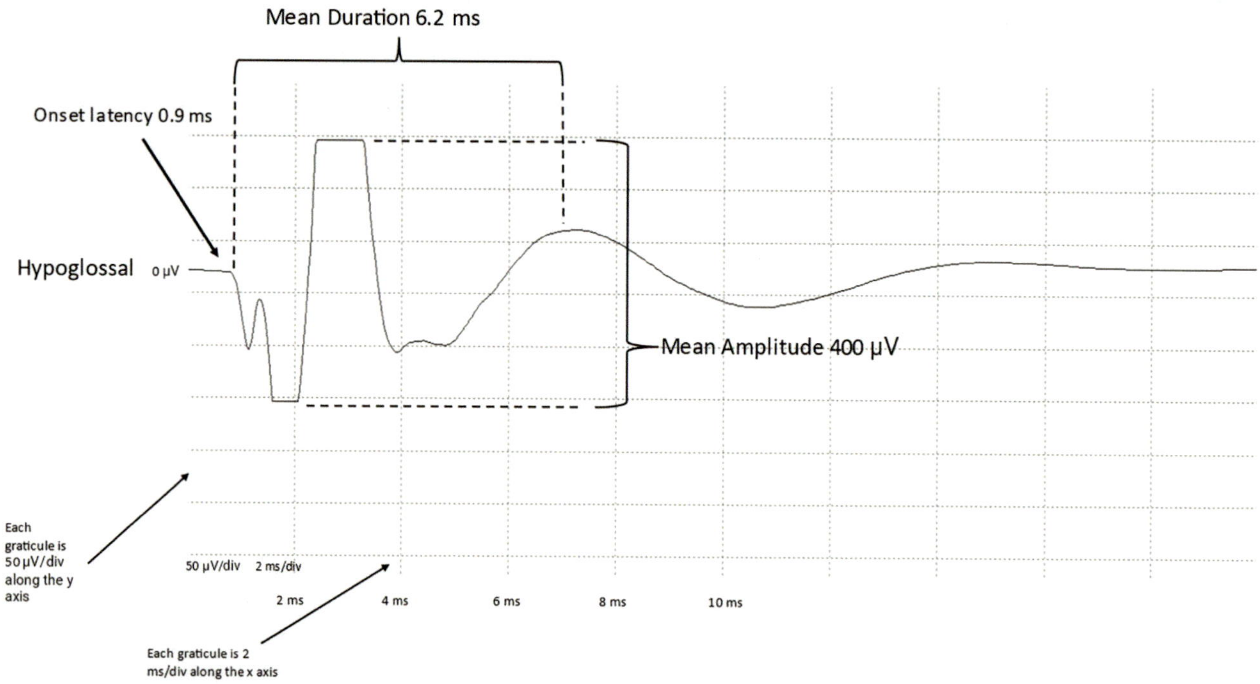


**Fig. 12.2** Direct stimulation of the hypoglossal nerve recording from the genioglossus muscle at a stimulation intensity of 2.0 mA

## Further Reading


Castilla-Garrido JM, Murgab-Oporto L. Intraoperative electro neurophysiological monitoring of basal cranial nerve surgery. Rev Neurol. 1999;11:573–82.

Duque CS, Londoño AF, Penagos AM, Urquijo DP, Dueñas JP. Hypoglossal nerve monitoring, a potential application of intraoperative nerve monitoring in head and neck surgery. World J Surg Oncol. 2013;11:225.

Randolph GW, Dralle H, Abdullah H, Barczynski M, Bellantone R, Brauckhoff M, et al. International Intraoperative Monitoring Study Group. Electrophysiologic recurrent laryngeal nerve monitoring during thyroid and parathyroid surgery: international standards guidelines statement. Laryngoscope. 2011;11:1–16.

Skinner SA. Neurophysiologic monitoring of the spinal accessory nerve, hypoglossal nerve and the spinomedullary region. J Clin Neurophysiol. 2011;11(6):587–98.

Walshe P, Shandilya M, Rowley H, Zahrovich A, Walsh RM, Walsh M, et al. Use of intra-operative nerve stimulator in identifying the hypoglossal nerve. J Laryngol Otol. 2006;11:185–7.

# 13 Intraoperative Neurophysiological Monitoring for the Phrenic Nerve: Case Illustrations

Joseph DiAngelo, Pedro Garcia, Thomas Lopazanski, Alan D. Deutsch, and Alexander L. Shifrin

The phrenic nerves originate from the anterior rami of the third through fifth cervical nerve roots bilaterally and supply motor innervation to the diaphragms. Injury to the phrenic nerve can result in paralysis of the ipsilateral diaphragm, leading to symptoms of dyspnea. As a portion of the phrenic nerve travels through the neck, there is a potential for injury to the nerve during the radical neck dissection. The phrenic nerve is monitored by using a single long 19 mm subdermal needle electrode (Rochester disposable Horizon subdermal needle electrode®; LifeSync Neuro; Coral Springs, FL) placed at the level of the diaphragm. A second reference needle electrode is placed at the xiphoid area of the sternum. A Prass monopolar cathode stimulator probe (Medtronic Xomed Inc.®; Minneapolis, MN) is used by the surgeon to directly stimulate and identify the phrenic nerve. A reference stimulator anode electrode is placed in the ipsilateral trapezius muscle. Stimulus intensities of 3.0–8.0 milliamps (mA) are used. All waveforms and data were obtained utilizing Cadwell Cascade® (Kennewick, WA) intraoperative monitoring recording equipment (Figs. 13.1 and 13.2).

J. DiAngelo · P. Garcia · T. Lopazanski · A. D. Deutsch
Monmouth Ocean Neurology, Neptune, NJ, USA

A. L. Shifrin (✉)
Surgical Director of Endocrinology, Atlantic Health CentraState Medical Center, Freehold, NJ, USA


A. L. Shifrin et al. (eds.), *Atlas of Intraoperative Cranial Nerve Monitoring in Thyroid and Head and Neck Surgery*,
https://doi.org/10.1007/978-3-031-24613-5_13

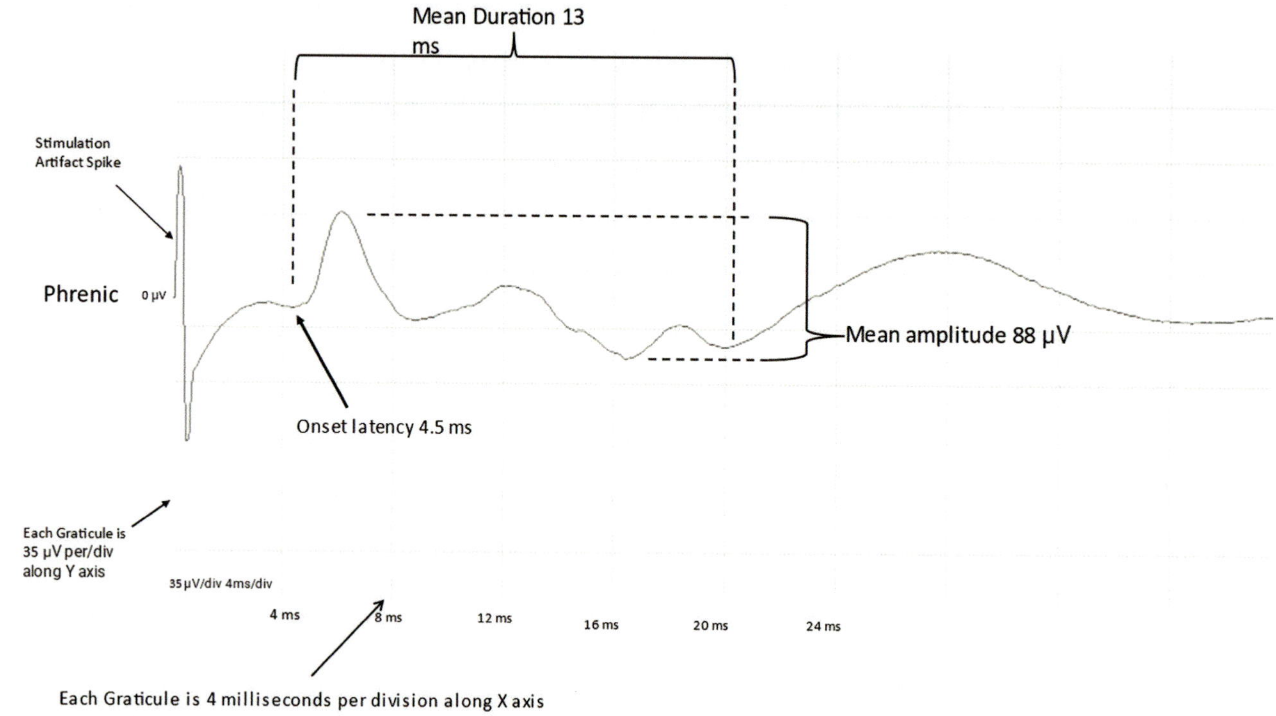


**Fig. 13.1** Direct stimulation of the phrenic nerve at a stimulus intensity of 4 mA

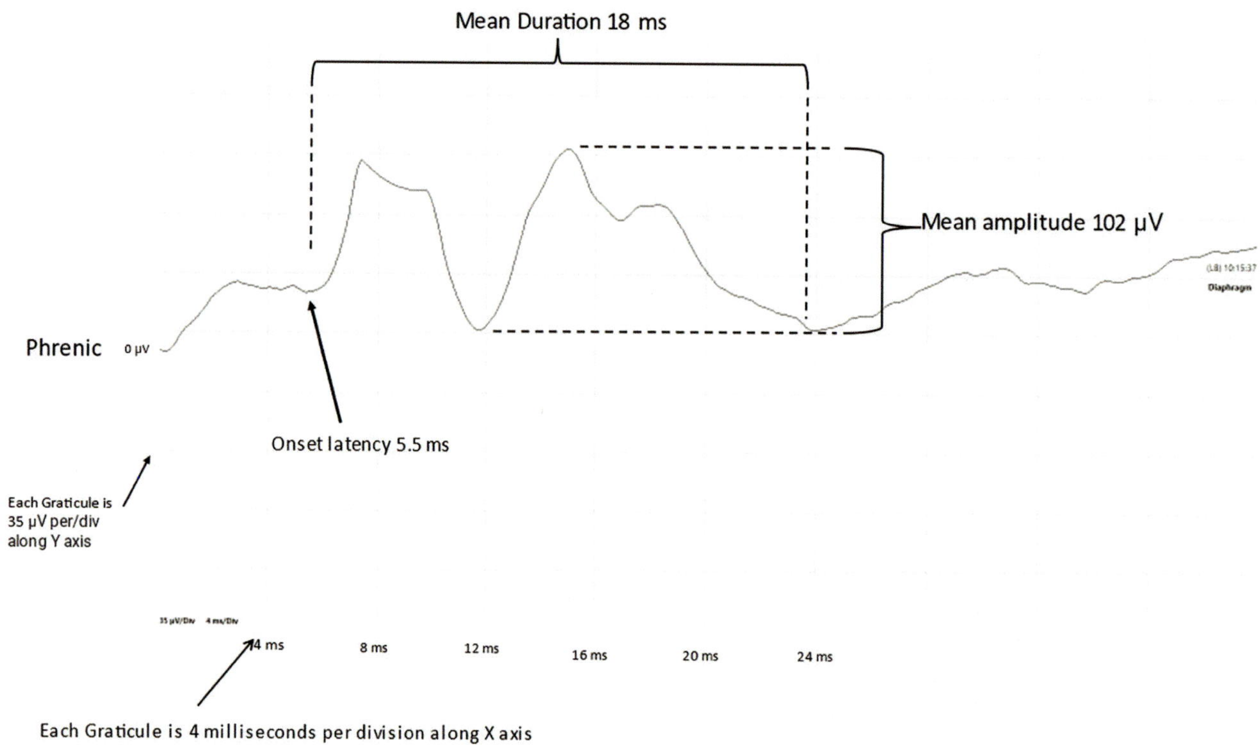


**Fig. 13.2** Direct stimulation of the phrenic nerve at a stimulus intensity of 3.0 mA

## Further Reading

Grande-Martín A, Martínez-Moreno A, Sánchez-Honrubia R, Pardal-Fernández J. Intraoperative neurophysiological monitoring of the phrenic nerve: utility and descriptions of the technique. Innov Surg Tech. 2019;97(2):103–7.

Mazzoni M, Solinas C, Sisillo E, Bortone F, Susini G. Intraoperative phrenic nerve monitoring in cardiac surgery. Chest. 1996;109(6):1455–60.

Sánchez-Honrubia RM, Pardal-Fernández JM. Intraoperative neurophysiological monitoring of the phrenic nerve: utility and descriptions of the technique. Cir Esp. 2019;97(2):103–7. https://doi.org/10.1016/j.ciresp.2018.11.002. Epub 2018 Dec 20. PMID: 30580833.

# 14 Continuous Intraoperative Neuromonitoring in Thyroid Surgery

Rick Schneider and Che-Wei Wu

## Introduction

Intraoperative neural monitoring (IONM) is becoming increasingly common in thyroid surgery. Strict standardization and quality control, as well as technical improvements, have resulted in sensitivities above 90%, suggesting that IONM is good enough to detect the recurrent laryngeal nerve (RLN) dysfunction and predict postoperative vocal cord (VC) palsy.

With the introduction of continuous IONM (CIONM), the functionality of the entire vagus nerve (VN)-RLN axis can be continuously monitored during thyroid surgery to alert the surgeon to dangerous maneuvers and allow for nerve recovery [1]. Several clinical data demonstrate no disadvantages associated with circular dissection of the VN segment or continuous stimulation per se. Moreover, elderly patients with advanced AV block and/or pacemakers or even children can be safely monitored [2, 3]. As noted in a proof-a-concept study, CIONM resulted in parasympathetic dominance that was not offset by increased sympathetic activity. The increased parasympathetic tone did not affect cardiac or hemodynamic parameters or levels of the proinflammatory cytokine TNF-α [4]. To facilitate the interpretation of clinically important quantitative electromyograms, so-called unfavorable combined electromyography (EMG) events (amplitude decrease <50%, latency increase >10%) were defined as indicative of impending traction-related damage to the RLN. If not responded to, these combined events can lead to loss of electromyographic (EMG) signal, a serious and barely reversible condition [5]. An intraoperative amplitude recovery of ≥50% from baseline reliably predicts normal early postoperative VC function after transient signal loss. The predictive accuracy of continuous stimulation is very high at 99.5% and provides a perfect basis for intraoperative decision-making for or against contralateral surgery. If signal loss persists or intraoperative recovery of EMG amplitude on the first resection side is less than 50%, a staged approach should be established to protect these patients from the serious postoperative complication of bilateral VC palsy [6, 7].

As recently shown, CIONM reduced early postoperative and permanent VC palsy compared with intermittent IONM alone [8]. To achieve optimal predictive power, the L1, V1, R1, R2, V2, L2 concept of the INMSG and troubleshooting algorithm for loss of EMG signal must be followed [9]. Under this premise, the CIONM achieves a sensitivity of 90.9%, specificity of 99.7%, positive predictive value of 88.2%, and negative predictive value of 99.8% [8].

## Prerequisites for CIONM

### Evaluation of VC Movement

For correct interpretation, intraoperative EMG findings must be correlated with VC function. Laryngoscopy is an essential part of the preoperative examination in thyroid surgery (L1).

### Concept of the Dominant Side

In planned bilateral thyroid surgery, the dominant side is the larger lobe or the lobe containing the suspected or proven lesion or hyperfunctional nodule that is the indication for surgery. In multinodular goiter, the dominant lobe is usually

R. Schneider (✉)
Department of Visceral, Vascular and Endocrine Surgery, University Hospital, Martin Luther University Halle-Wittenberg, Halle (Saale), Germany
e-mail: rick.schneider@uk-halle.de

C.-W. Wu
Department of Otorhinolaryngology-Head and Neck Surgery, Kaohsiung Medical University Hospital, Faculty of Medicine, College of Medicine, Kaohsiung Medical University, Kaohsiung, Taiwan
e-mail: cwwu@kmu.edu.tw


A. L. Shifrin et al. (eds.), *Atlas of Intraoperative Cranial Nerve Monitoring in Thyroid and Head and Neck Surgery*,
https://doi.org/10.1007/978-3-031-24613-5_14

not only larger but also has more nodules. The start of resection on the dominant side is directed toward the leading thyroid pathology responsible for most symptoms.

## Informed Consent

With regard to the treatment of their disease, patients are very interested in shared decision-making. Patient autonomy requires that the informed consent form specifies the use of CIONM and clarifies the need for a staged procedure in case of loss of EMG signal on the first side of resection.

## CIONM Equipment

It is performed with the following commercially available devices:

- hand-held monopolar stimulator probe (4 pulses/s, 100 μs, 1 mA; Medtronic) for intermittent IONM,
- the automatic periodic stimulation (APS) electrode (2.0 or 3.0 mm; Medtronic) for CIONM,
- noninvasive surface electrodes embedded or inked on the endotracheal tube (NIM EMG Endotracheal Tube; Medtronic) to contact with vocal cord for evoked EMG signal recording, and
- nerve monitoring systems (NIM Vital; Medtronic) with a pulse generator for continuous stimulation (1 Hz, 100 μs, 1 mA) and an EMG amplifier.

## Anesthesia and Endotracheal Tube Positioning

Monitored thyroid surgery is performed under general anesthesia, using the short-acting muscle relaxants to facilitate tracheal intubation and avoid prolonged neuromuscular block. The endotracheal tube is inserted under visual control or video laryngoscope to ensure correct placement of the recording surface electrode at the level of the VC [9]. Maintenance of an electrode impedance of <5 kΩ with an imbalance of <1 kΩ indicates optimal electrode-mucosal contact according to recently published guidelines for neural monitoring standards [7, 10].

## Procedure

To obtain meaningful EMG signals, the following points must be observed:

1. Collar incision, ranging from small incisions to extensive Kocher incisions.
2. Opening the carotid sheath at the level of the thyroid cartilage through a short incision, the length of which depends on the dimensions of the continuous stimulating electrode, and identifying the VN before exposing the thyroid gland through an anterior (midline) or lateral (between the sternohyoid and sternocleidomastoid) approach (Figs. 14.1 and 14.2). The VN most commonly courses medially and posteriorly (73%) and less commonly medially (15%), laterally (8%), or anteriorly (4%) to the internal jugular vein and common carotid artery [11]. The central approach is suitable for small, benign goiters, whereas the lateral approach, which allows greater exposure, is more appropriate for large goiters and reoperations. If the electrical wires can be routed outside the surgical field, the risk of accidental dislocation of the vagus electrode is much lower.
3. Morphological and functional examination of the VN with the hand-held IONM probe (4.0 Hz, 100 μs, 1 mA) (Figs. 14.3 and 14.4) before attaching the CIONM electrode to the nerve. If stimulation remains unsuccessful, the troubleshooting algorithm for IONM [2] must be followed. The right VN should be stimulated further down the neck to rule out the presence of a nonrecurrent inferior laryngeal nerve (1.4%) [12].
4. Circumferential dissection of a short segment (<1 cm) of the VN while preserving its blood supply (Figs. 14.5 and 14.6). The VN is enormously robust to the usual careful and meticulous surgical technique in the neck.
5. Placement of the APS electrode on the VN with initial stimulation at 1 mA and 1 Hz in a position where it cannot interfere with subsequent resection. The electrode has to be carefully positioned on the nerve at a 45-degree angle with the tabs of the housing held open with forceps and resting on the nerve (Fig. 14.7).
6. Calibration of the IONM system. After connecting the APS electrode to the NIM Vital nerve monitoring system, the baselines for latency and amplitude will be automatically calibrated (Fig. 14.8). For stable and reliable EMG signals, the baseline amplitude should reach ≥500 μV [17]. When the baseline amplitude is less than 500 μV, the anesthesiologist should position the endotracheal tube to achieve a waveform >500 μV. To optimize sensitivity to impending nerve injury, the baseline amplitude should be maximized.
7. Start CIONM and stimulation of the VN with the handheld intermittent nerve stimulation (V1) (Fig. 14.9). All subsequent EMG changes are measured against the calibrated amplitude and latency baselines and displayed on the screen as a function of time (Fig. 14.10). Audible and visual alarms can also be defined at thresholds that signal impending nerve injury and require release of the affected nerve. An upper limit for latency and a lower limit for amplitude were displayed as separate alarm

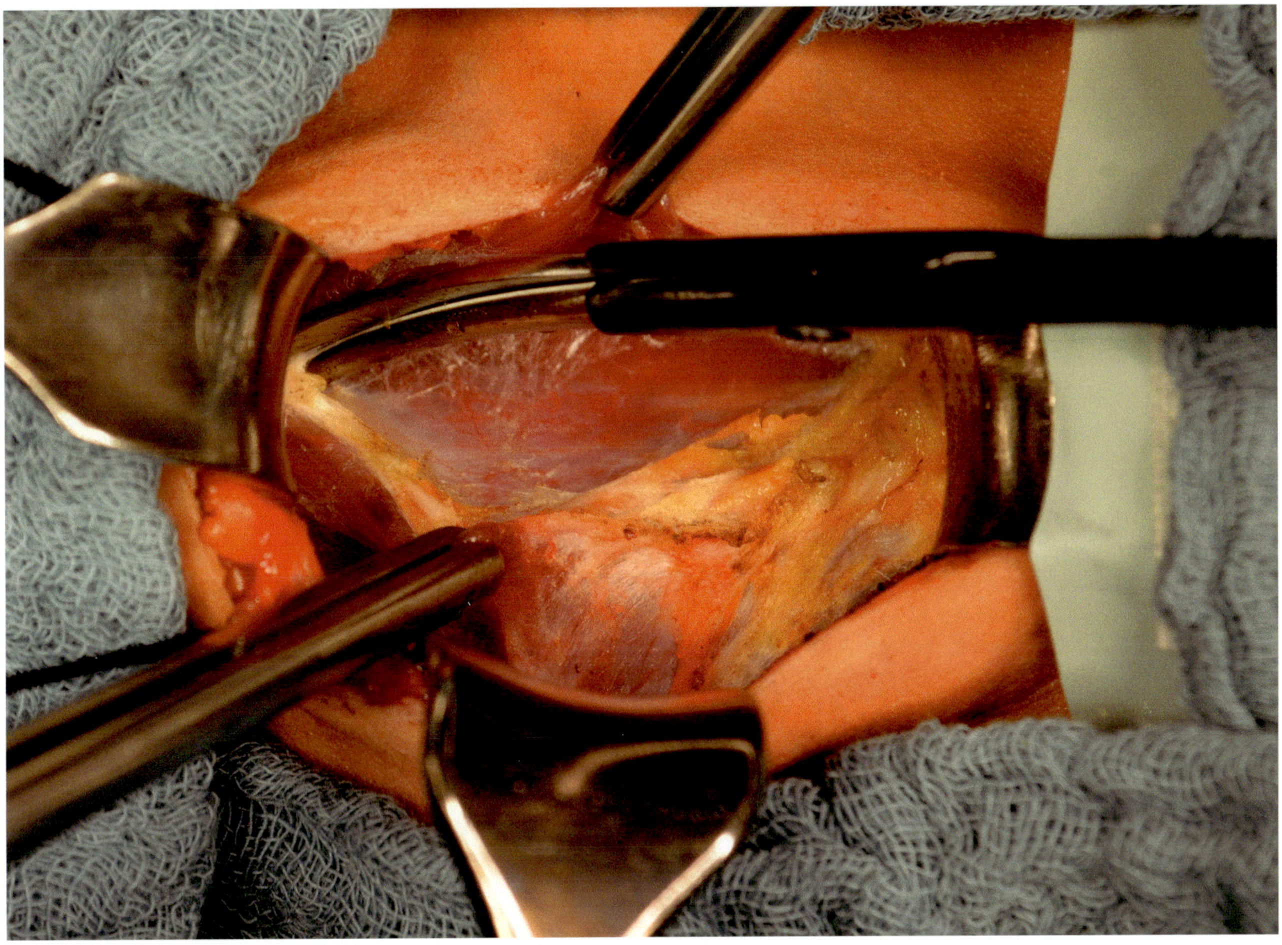

**Fig. 14.1** Medial approach after collar incision with dissection of the short straight neck muscle from the right thyroid capsule

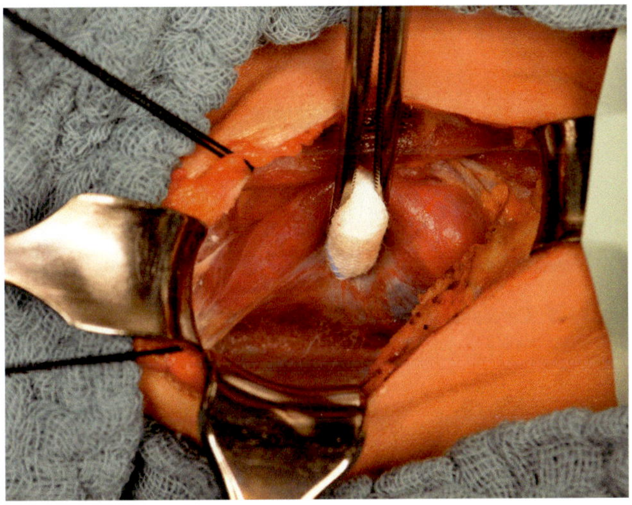

**Fig. 14.2** Complete mobilization of the short neck muscles laterally, medialization of the right thyroid lobe, and exposition of the carotid sheath

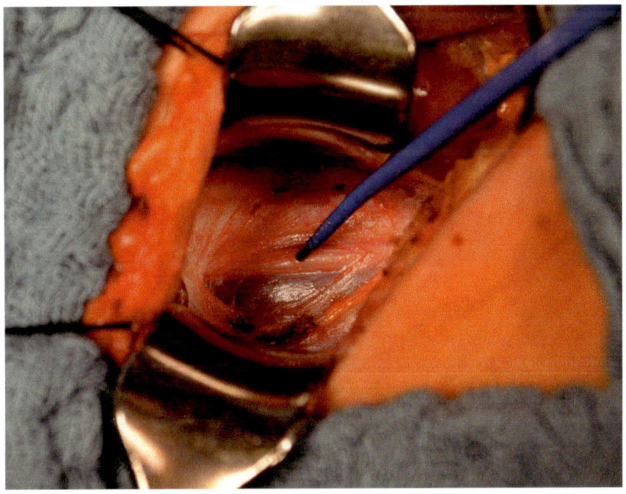

**Fig. 14.3** Opening the carotid sheath at the level of the thyroid cartilage through a short incision, the length of which depends on the dimensions of the stimulating electrode, and identifying the vagus nerve. Morphological and functional examination of the vagus nerve with the hand-held intermittent nerve stimulation probe before attaching the CIONM electrode to the nerve

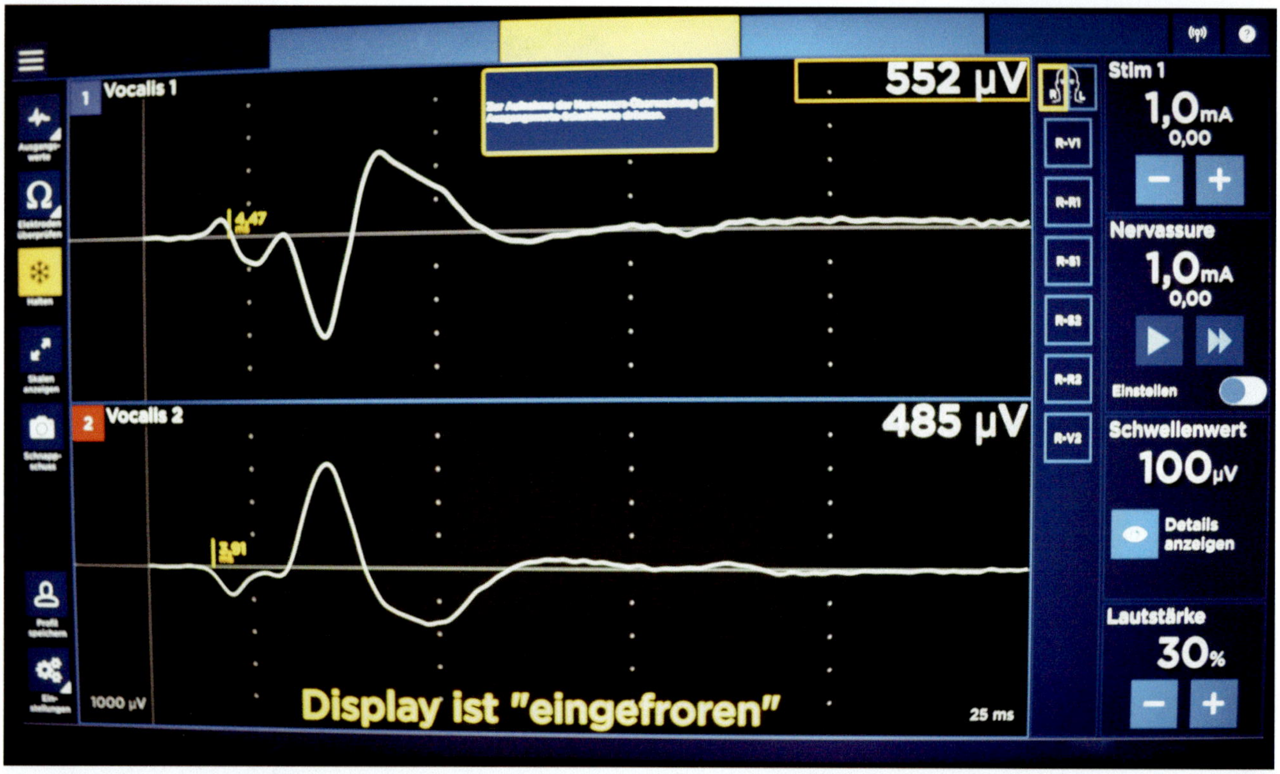


**Fig. 14.4** Monitor screen with normal EMG of the right vagus nerve as setup check

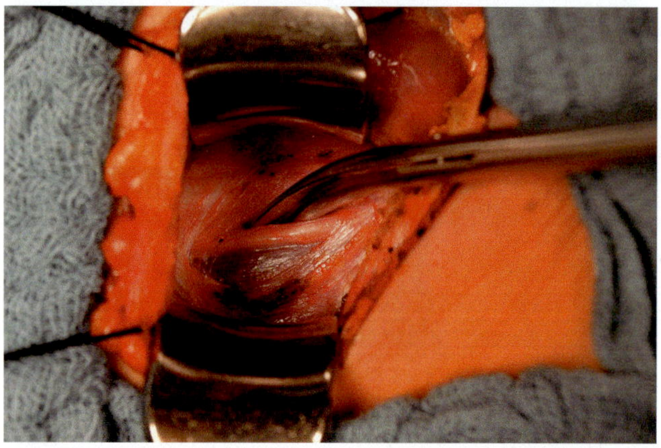

**Fig. 14.5** Circumferential dissection of a short segment (<1 cm) of the vagus nerve while preserving its blood supply. The vagus nerve is enormously robust to the usual careful and meticulous surgical technique in the neck

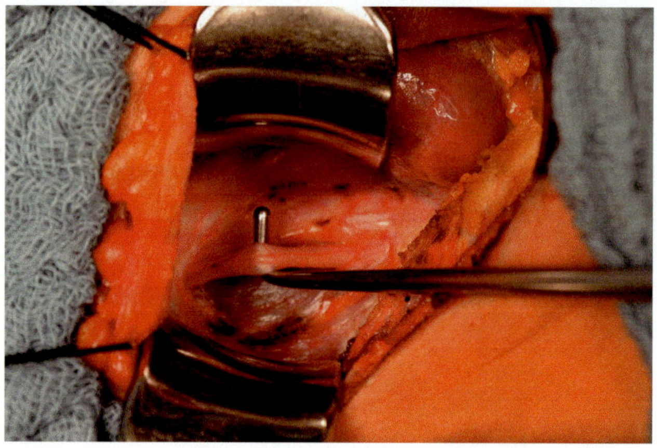

**Fig. 14.6** Careful elevation of the vagus nerve by driving under it with the nerve hook

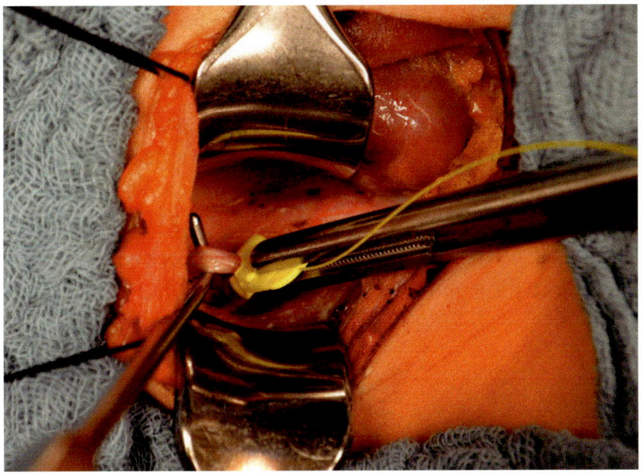

**Fig. 14.7** Placement of the APS electrode on the vagus nerve at a 45-degree angle with the tabs of the housing held open with forceps and resting on the nerve

lines. After establishing the APS baseline for amplitude and latency of the evoked response, continuous and intermittent stimulated EMG signals will be recorded.

8. In addition to CIONM with the APS electrode, the hand-held probe can be used for intermittent direct nerve stimulation by the surgeon to facilitate identification of the RLN (R1) (Figs. 14.11 and 14.12) and performance of the procedure. Dissection of the thyroid lobes is usually performed in a caudal to cranial direction with close observation of the course of the RLN. For larger retrosternal goiters, the upper pole can be mobilized first to expose the retrosternal portion of the goiter. After dissection of the thyroid lobe, the hand-held probe helps to monitor and confirm the final RLN function (R2) (Figs. 14.13 and 14.14).
9. At the end of surgery before removal of the APS electrode, the VN nerve is stimulated with the hand-held

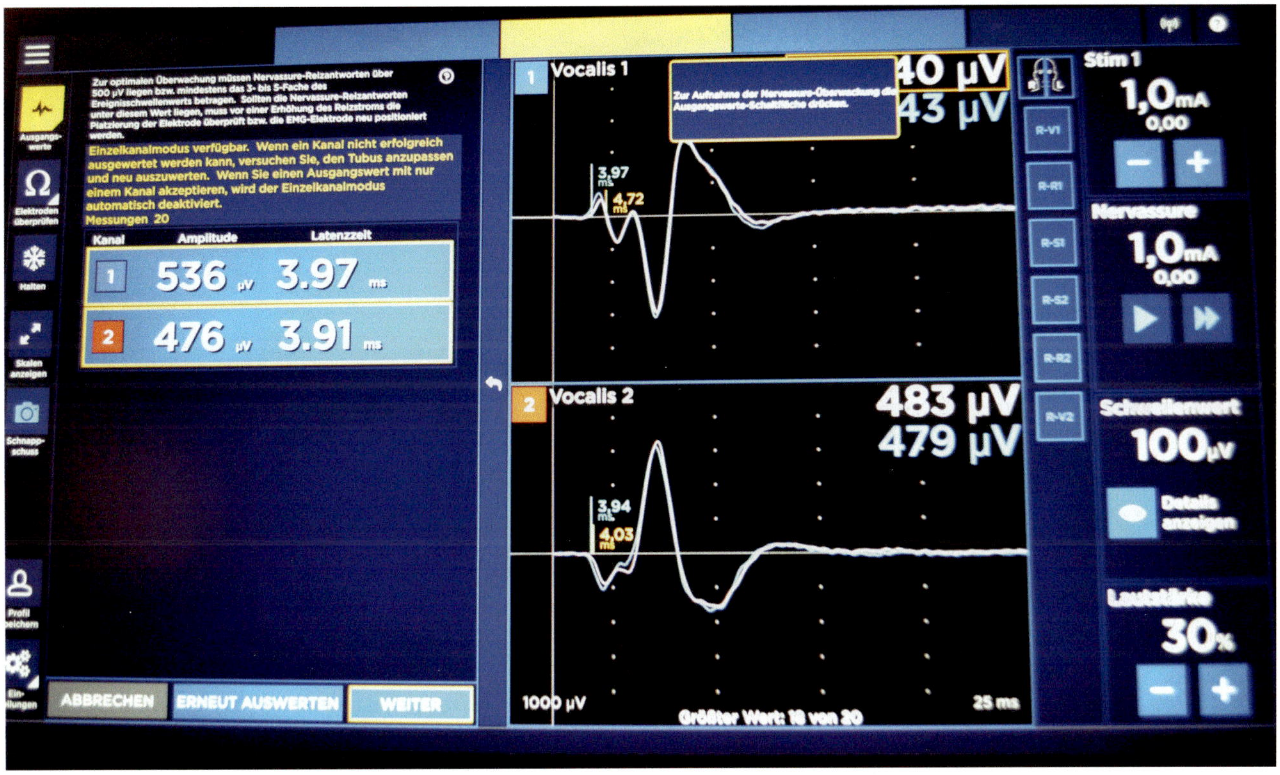


**Fig. 14.8** Calibration of the IONM system. After connecting the APS electrode to the NIM vital nerve monitoring system, the baselines for latency and amplitude were automatically calibrated. For stable and reliable EMG signals, the baseline amplitude should reach ≥500 µV

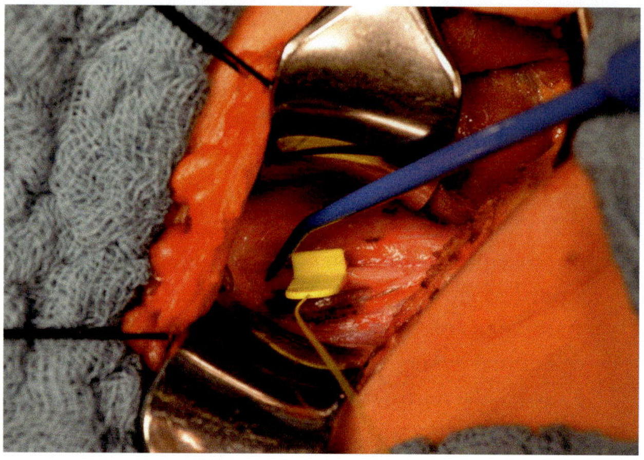

**Fig. 14.9** Start CIONM and stimulation of the vagus nerve with the hand-held intermittent nerve stimulation (V1)

intermittent nerve stimulation probe proximal (V2) (Figs. 14.15 and 14.16) to the electrode contact site to rule out electrode-induced segmental VN injury. EMG documentation is required in the patient's medical records and includes time-traceable measurements of V1, R1, R2, and V2 for each side.

10. Postoperative laryngeal examination (L2) is important to improve the prognostic correlation between CIONM stimulation and postoperative VC function.

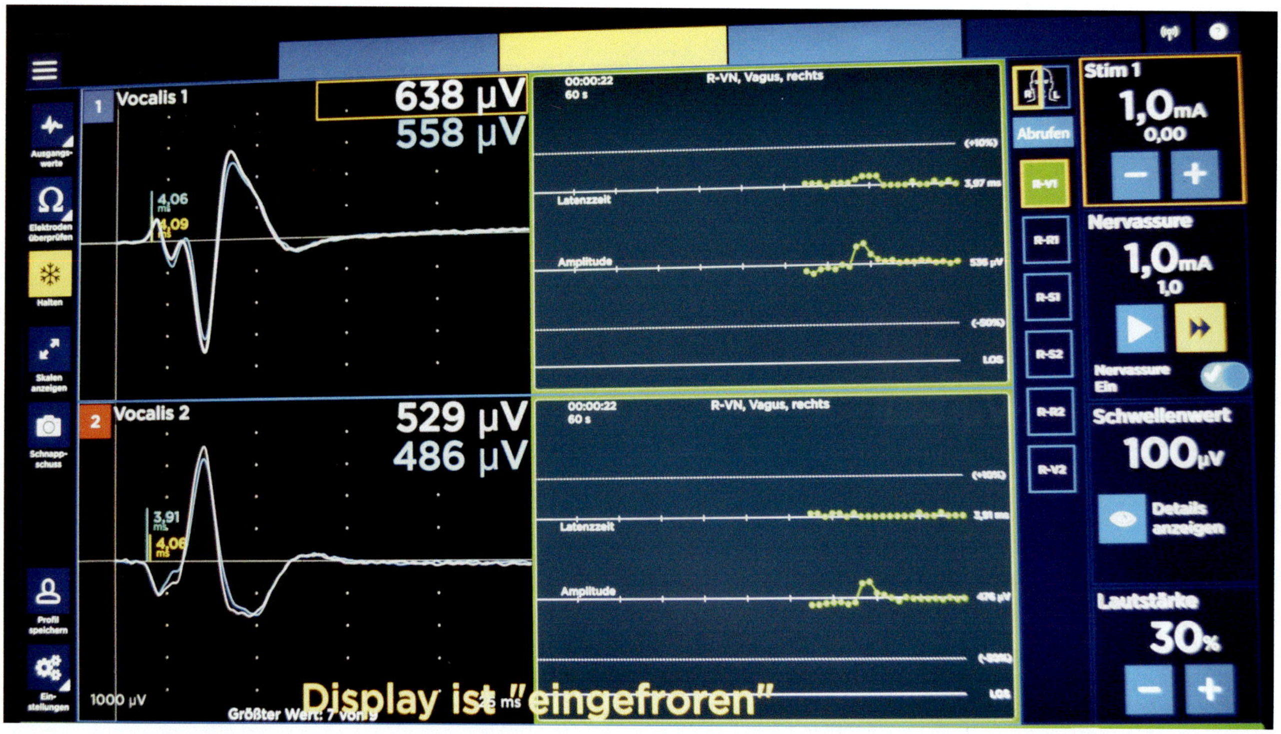


**Fig. 14.10** Monitor screen with normal EMG of the right vagus nerve (left side). All subsequent EMG changes are measured against the calibrated amplitude and latency baselines and displayed on the screen as a function of time (right side). Audible and visual alarms can also be defined at thresholds that signal impending nerve injury and require release of the affected nerve. An upper limit for latency and a lower limit for amplitude were displayed as separate alarm lines

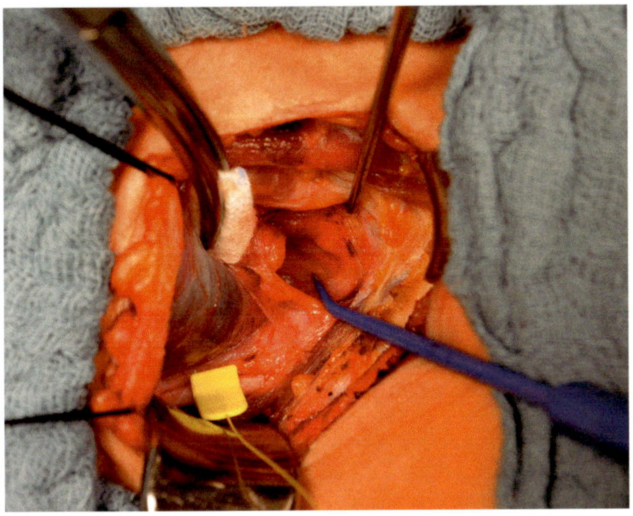

**Fig. 14.11** Mapping and identification using the hand-held probe with intermittent direct nerve stimulation (R1)

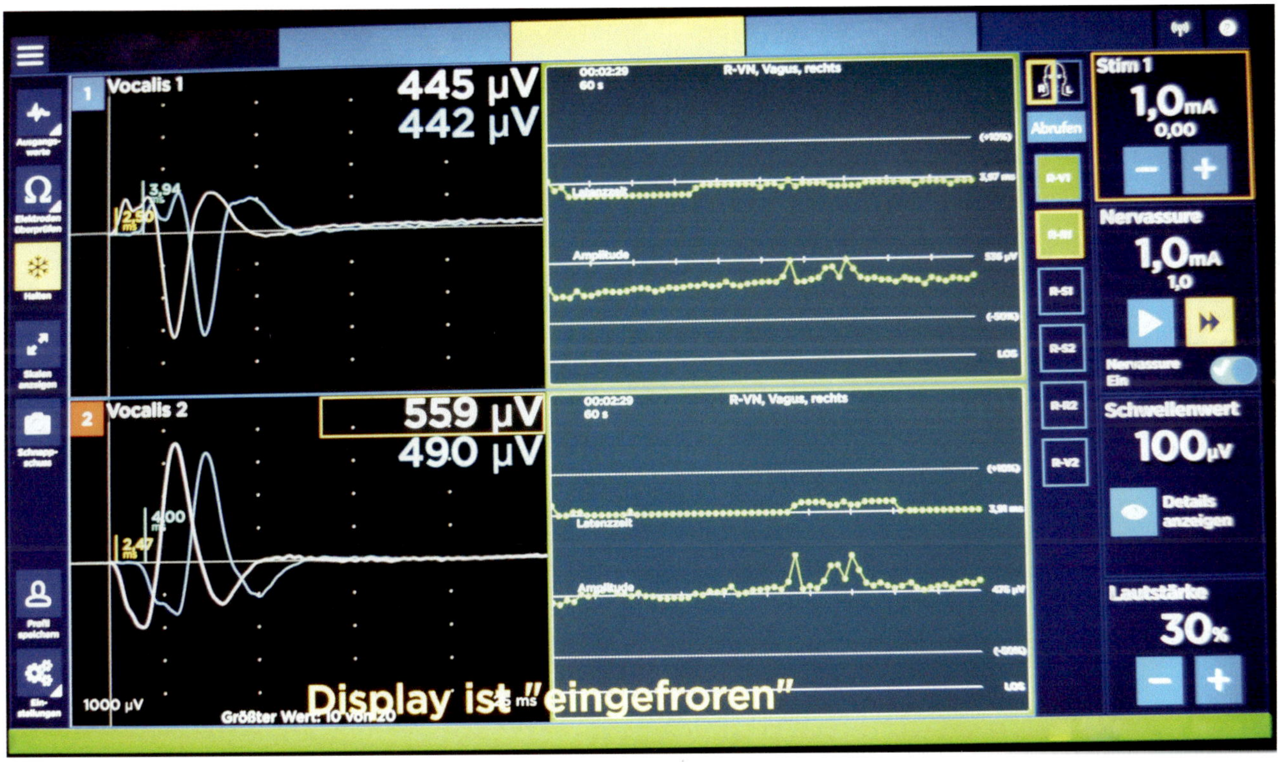


**Fig. 14.12** Monitor screen with normal EMG of the right recurrent laryngeal nerve (white EMG) (R1) and the right vagus nerve (blue EMG)

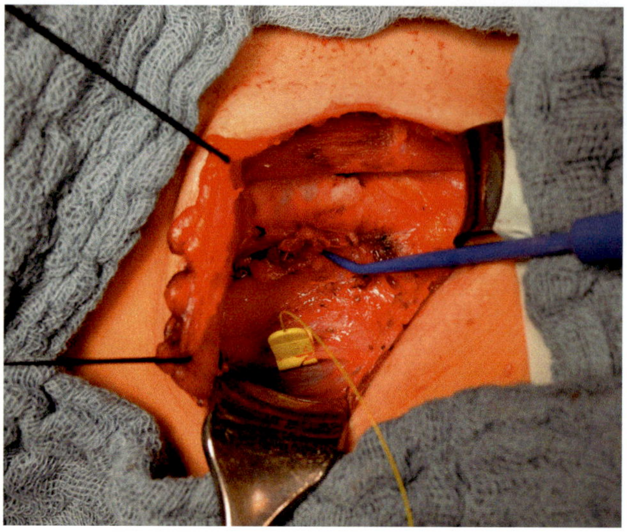

**Fig. 14.13** After dissection of the thyroid lobe, the hand-held probe helps monitor final RLN function (R2)

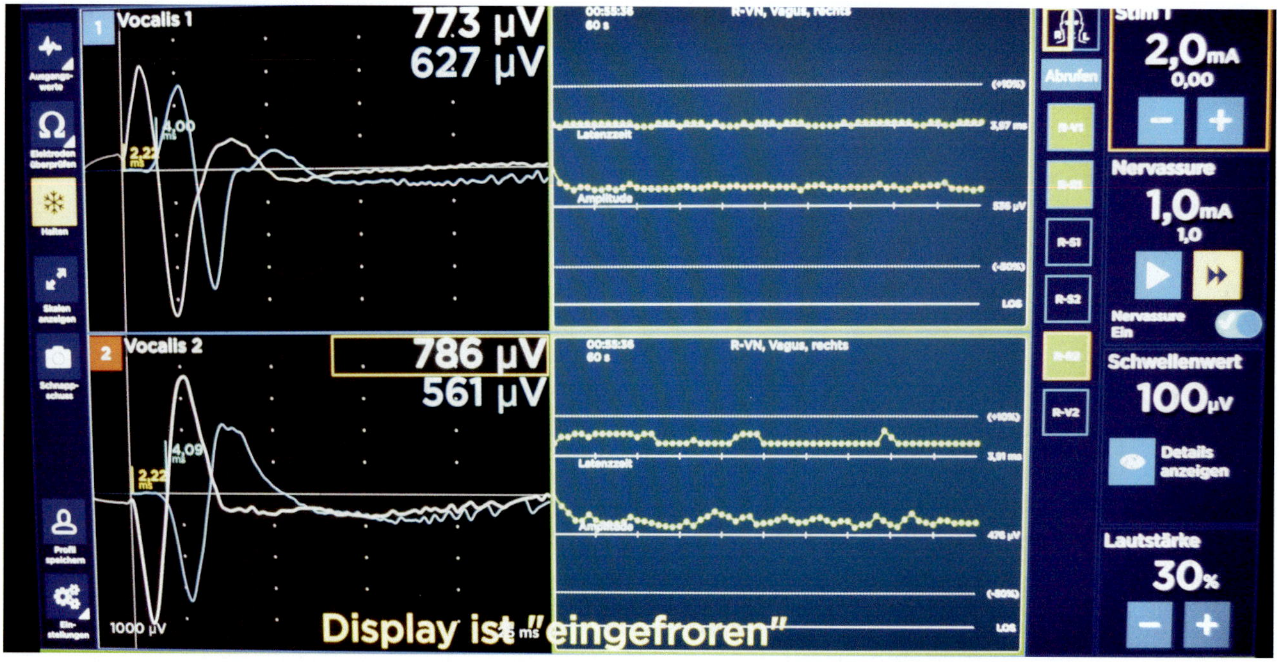


**Fig. 14.14** Monitor screen with normal EMG of the right recurrent laryngeal nerve (white EMG) (R2) and the right vagus nerve (blue EMG) after dissection

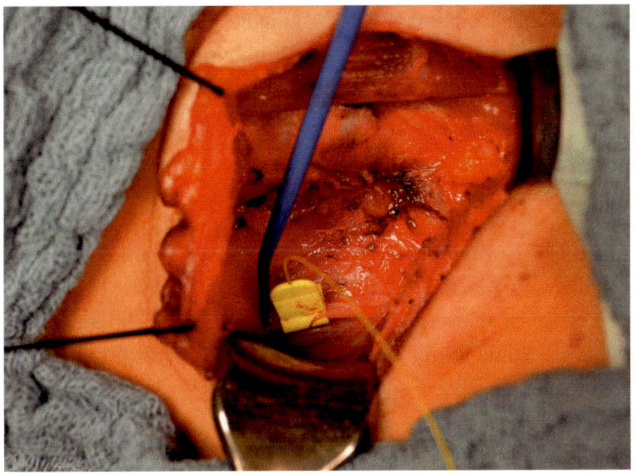

**Fig. 14.15** At the end of surgery before removal of the APS electrode, the VN nerve is stimulated with the hand-held intermittent nerve stimulation probe proximal (V2) to the electrode contact site to rule out electrode-induced segmental VN injury

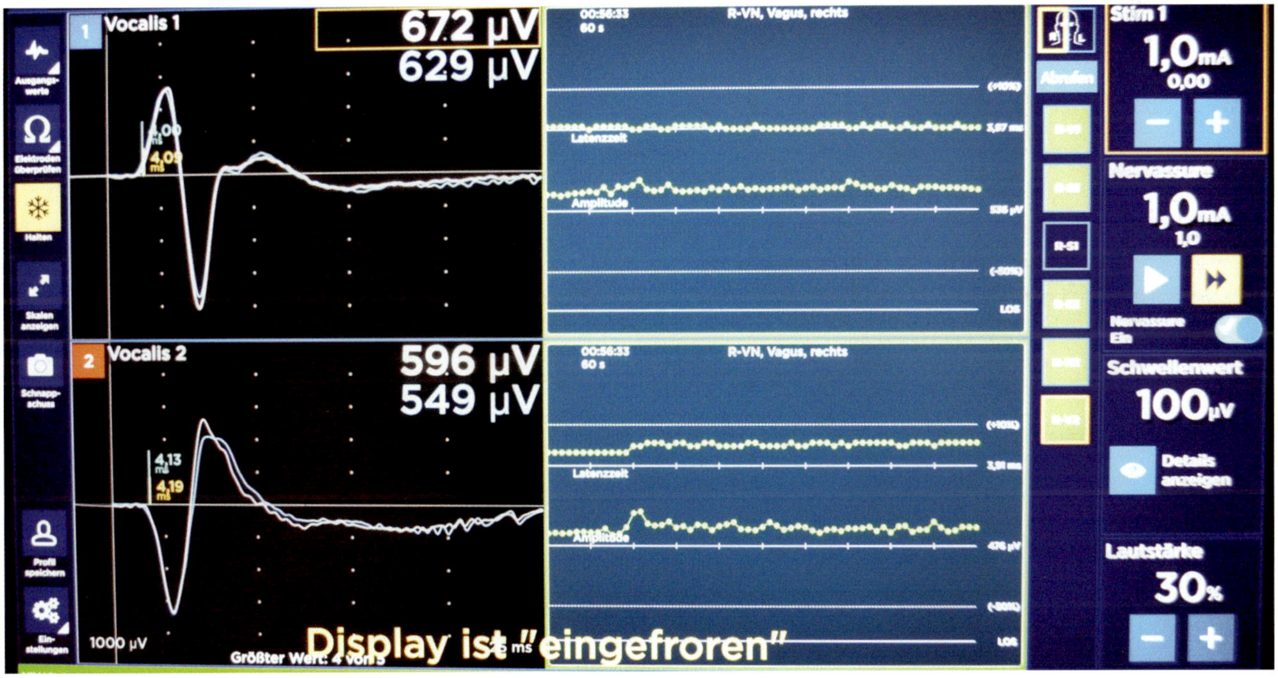


**Fig. 14.16** Monitor screen with normal EMG of the right vagus nerve after dissection (V2)

## Evaluation of EMG Data

### Impending Neuronal Damage

Skillful application of CIONM requires experience and observation of the EMG screen to facilitate interpretation of clinically relevant quantitative EMG signals from "normal" EMG (Fig. 14.17) leads. Unfavorable "combined" EMG events with specific concurrent changes in both signal amplitude and latency, defined as a decrease in amplitude of more than 50% and increase in latency of more than 10% compared with baseline values, indicate clinically important EMG thresholds indicative of impending nerve damage (Fig. 14.18).

### Artifacts

Periods of minor decrease or increase in amplitude or latency may occur more than once during CIONM. Repeated increases or decreases in both amplitude and latency may be artifactual, likely due to rotation or upward/downward

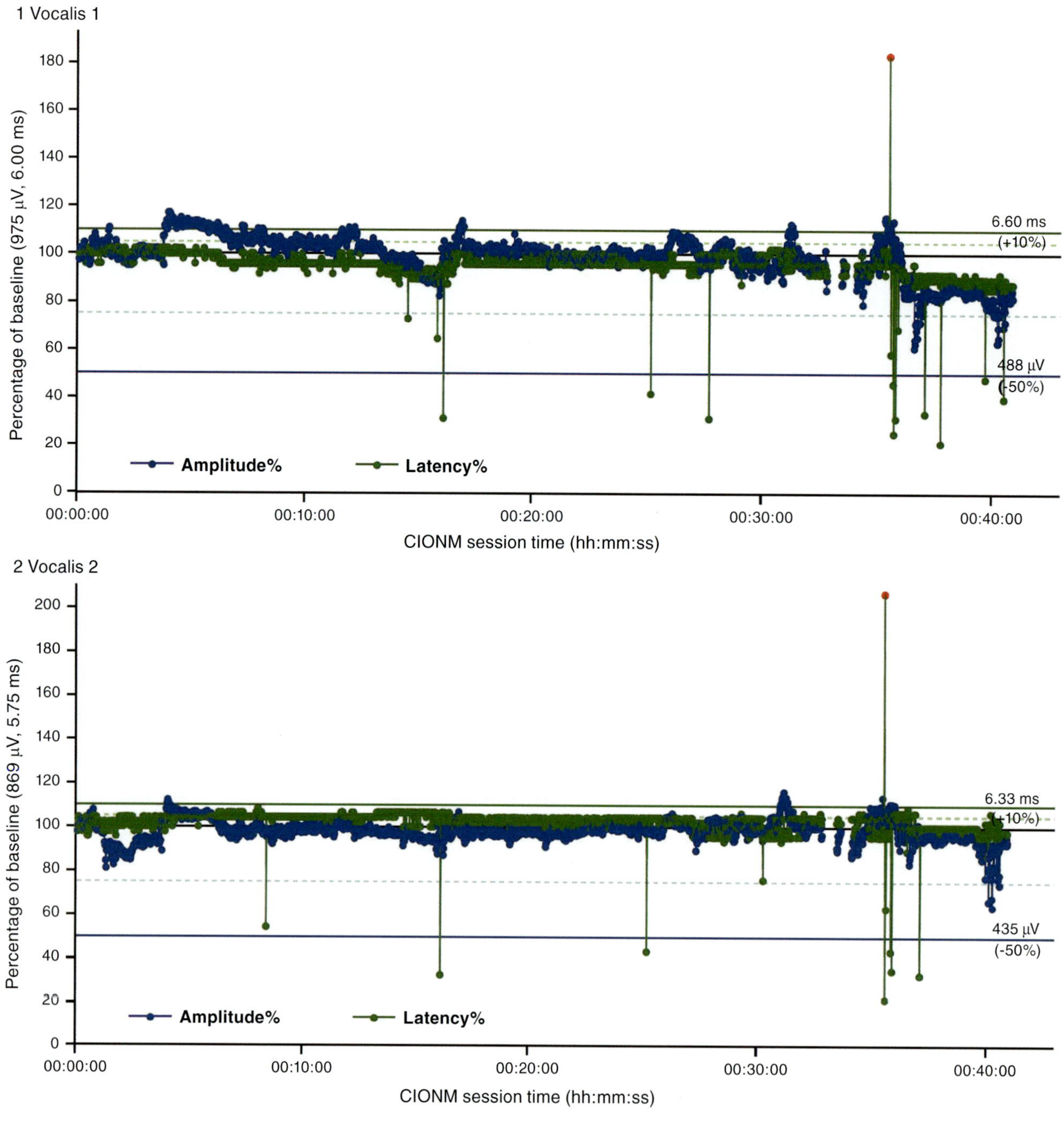


**Fig. 14.17** Uneventful EMG tracing during thyroid surgery on the left side

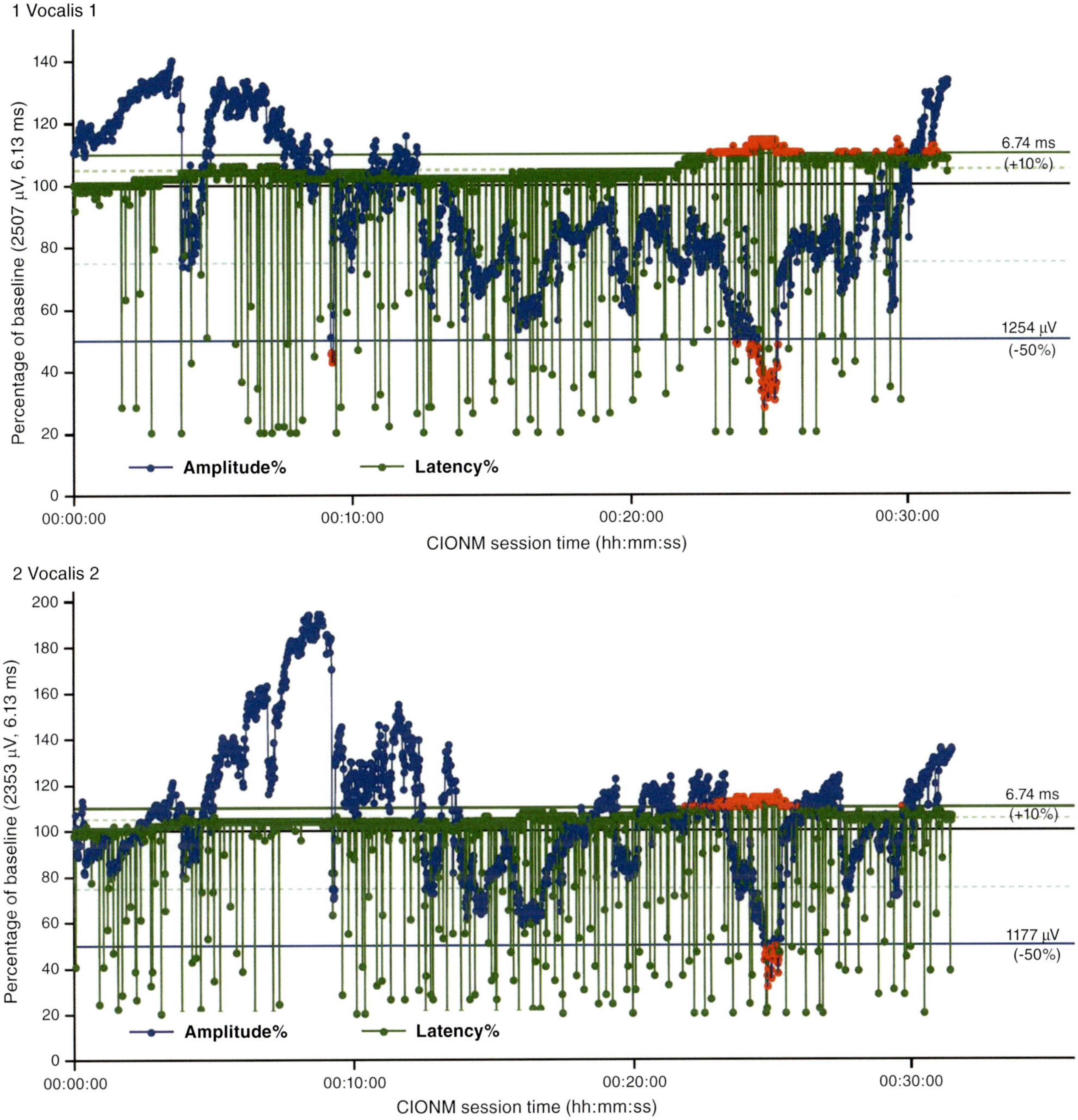


**Fig. 14.18** "Combined EMG event" during surgery on the left side. It is defined as a simultaneous decrease in amplitude by more than 50% of baseline and increase in latency by more than 10% of baseline. It is to be interpreted as a prodrome of an impending loss of signal. If the damaging maneuver (mainly traction) on the recurrent laryngeal nerve is stopped immediately, the combined event remains reversible and normal postoperative vocal cord function results

displacement of the EMG tube or tracheal shift with impaired contact between the recording electrodes and VC as a result of thyroid manipulation. In addition to transient loss of EMG recording due to coagulation with bipolar forceps, dislocation of the vagus electrode may occur after inadvertently pulling the lead wire; or a mismatch between the size of the VN and the electrode may result in poor stimulation characteristics. An "EMG storm" with repeated transient lapses in EMG recording followed by increased amplitude values is caused by poor vagus contact of an oversized vagus electrode. Typically, and in contrast to the dangerous traction-induced EMG changes, the harmless artifacts resolve after repositioning of the thyroid gland to its original position (Figs. 14.19, 14.20, and 14.21). Isolated amplitude or latency changes are not associated with VC palsy.

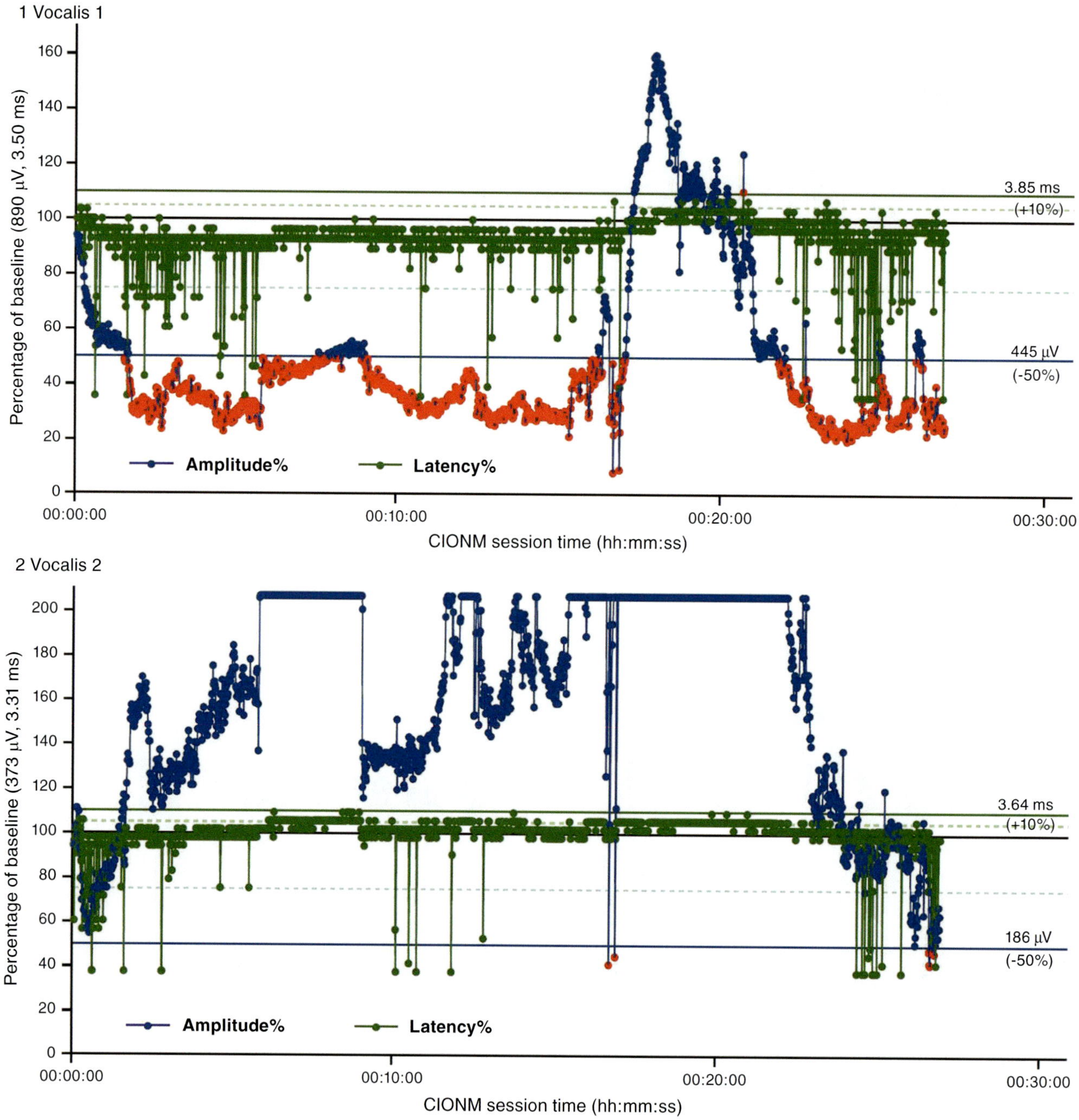


**Fig. 14.19** Artifactual isolated amplitude decrease during thyroid surgery on the right side. The amplitude drops occur only in one EMG channel, while in the second channel the amplitudes rise simultaneously above the level of the initial values. Causes may be horizontal or vertical tube dislocations. These EMG changes are not dangerous with normal postoperative vocal cord function

## Signal Recovery

Signal recovery of ≥50% of baseline nerve amplitude after loss of EMG signal always signifies normal postoperative VC function, whereas signal recovery <50% preceded early VC palsy in almost all patients with segmental type 1 injury and in two-thirds of patients with global type 2 injury, which is extremely important information for surgeons in planned bilateral operations (Figs. 14.22 and 14.23). Nerve function recovers completely after LOS within the first 15–20 min (segmental lesion type 1: 6.9–8.0 min; global lesion type 2: 13.0–15.6 min), which means that decision-making is possible after 20 min of waiting [6].

Because CIONM indicates impending nerve damage with an unfavorable condition that can reverse nerve damage as neuropraxia, it increases the accuracy of predicting VC function.

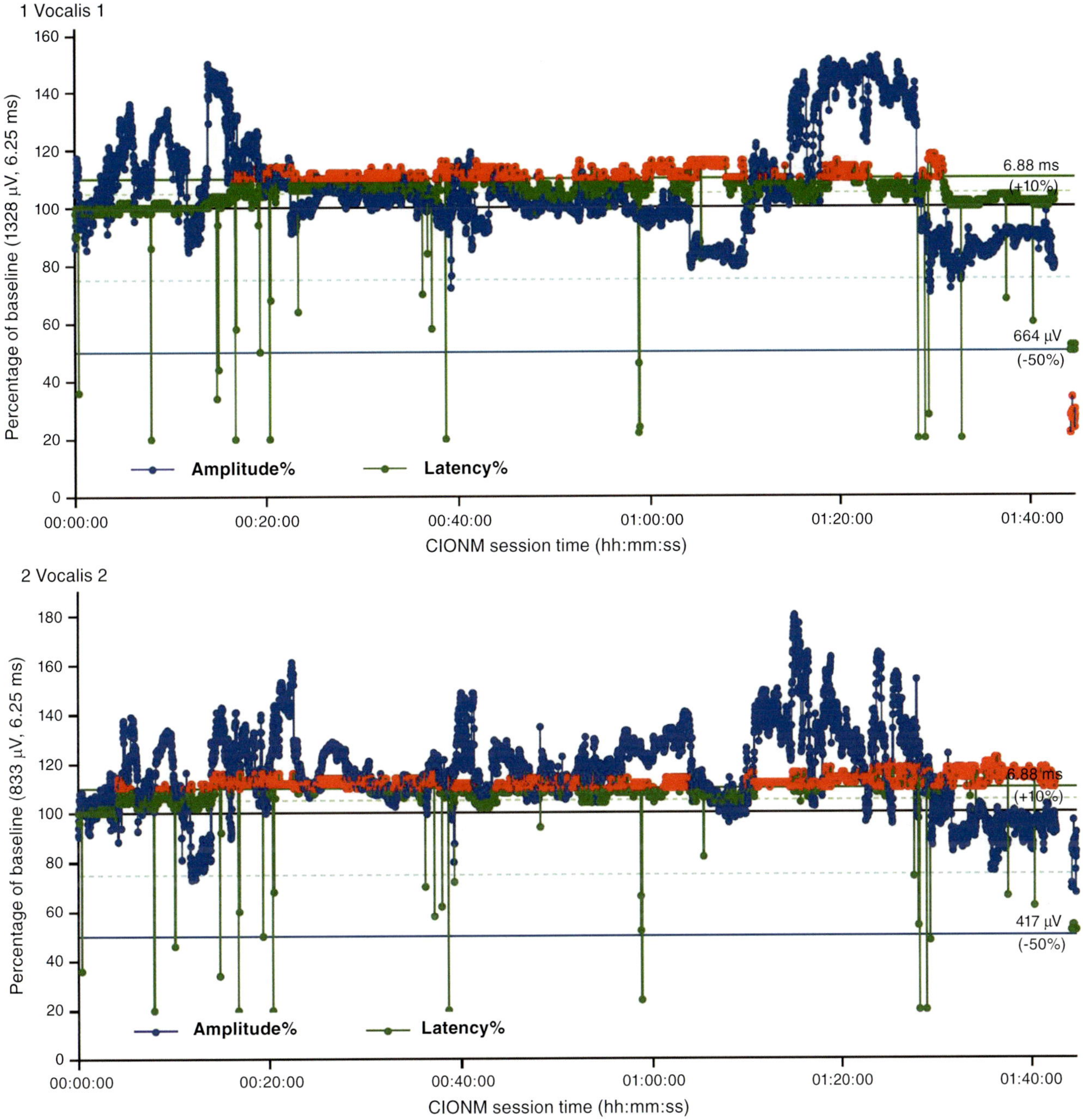


**Fig. 14.20** Artifactual isolated latency increase during thyroid surgery on the left side. The latency increase as a calculated EMG parameter is artifactual due to changes in EMG shape with displacement of the measurement point on the x-axis. The repeated change of the EMG shape with back-and-forth jumping of the latency is also called latency jumping. These EMG changes are not dangerous with normal postoperative vocal cord function

## Definite Loss of EMG Signal and Staged Thyroidectomy

The prediction accuracy of CIONM is very high at 99.5% and provides a perfect basis for intraoperative decision-making for or against contralateral surgery (Figs. 14.24 and 14.25). If loss of signal persists in a planned bilateral thyroidectomy or intraoperative recovery of EMG amplitude on the first resection side is less than 50%, a staged procedure should be decided to protect these patients from the serious postoperative complication of bilateral RLN palsy. A second staged thyroidectomy should be performed as a logical consequence after recovery of VC function.

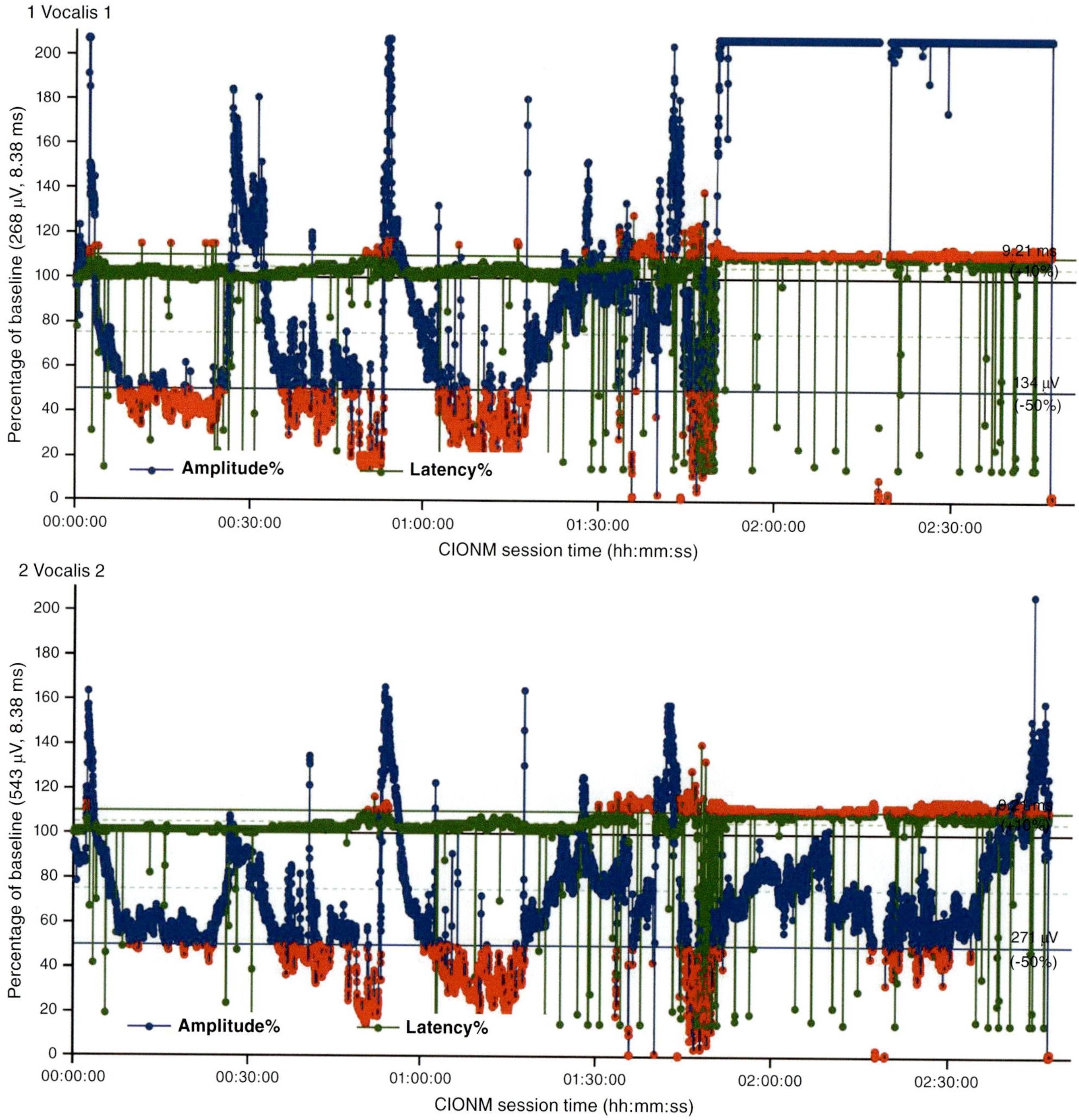


**Fig. 14.21** Artifactual repeated amplitude drops and latency increase during thyroid surgery on the left side. These EMG changes can be attributed to impaired contact between the tube adhesive electrode and the mucosa due to a tube that is too small or unfavorable anatomical conditions. Although these EMG changes are not dangerous, they significantly complicate the interpretation of actual pathological EMG changes. It results in normal postoperative vocal cord function

**Note**

All images are taken on the right side of the patient from an operating viewpoint. The patient's eyes are on the left edge of the image, the patient's feet on the right.

In all EMG tracing figures, the blue curve denotes nerve amplitude, whereas the green curve indicates latency. Both images (vocalis 1 and vocalis 2) result from the two pairs of recording electrodes of the EMG tube from the stimulated ipsilateral vocal muscle.

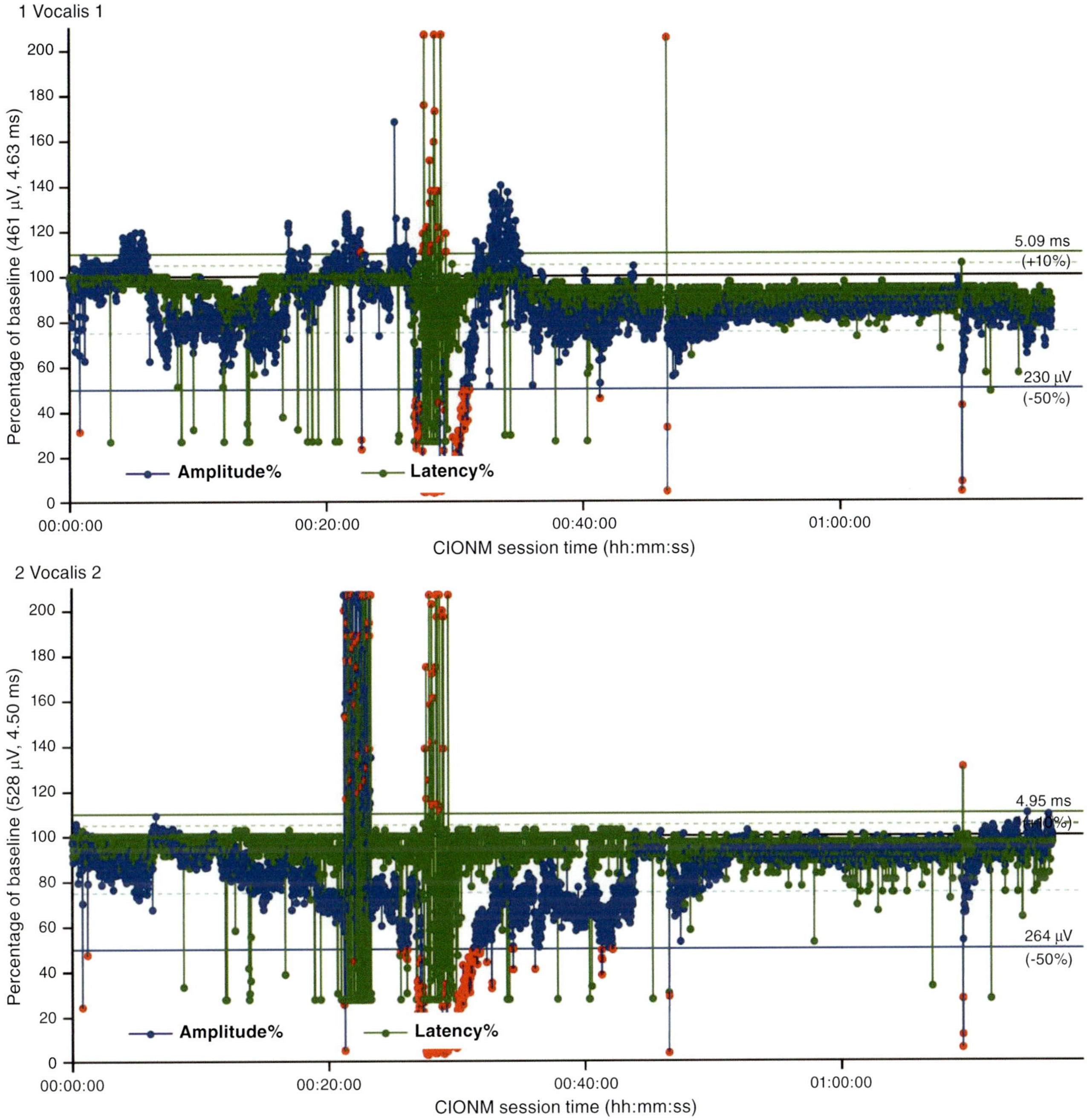


**Fig. 14.22** Transient segmental loss of signal (type 1) after mild clamping of the recurrent laryngeal nerve on the right side, in which the nerve monitoring signal is lost all of a sudden with drop of amplitude, and intraoperative recovery of EMG signal with amplitude recovery >50% of baseline and normal postoperative vocal cord function

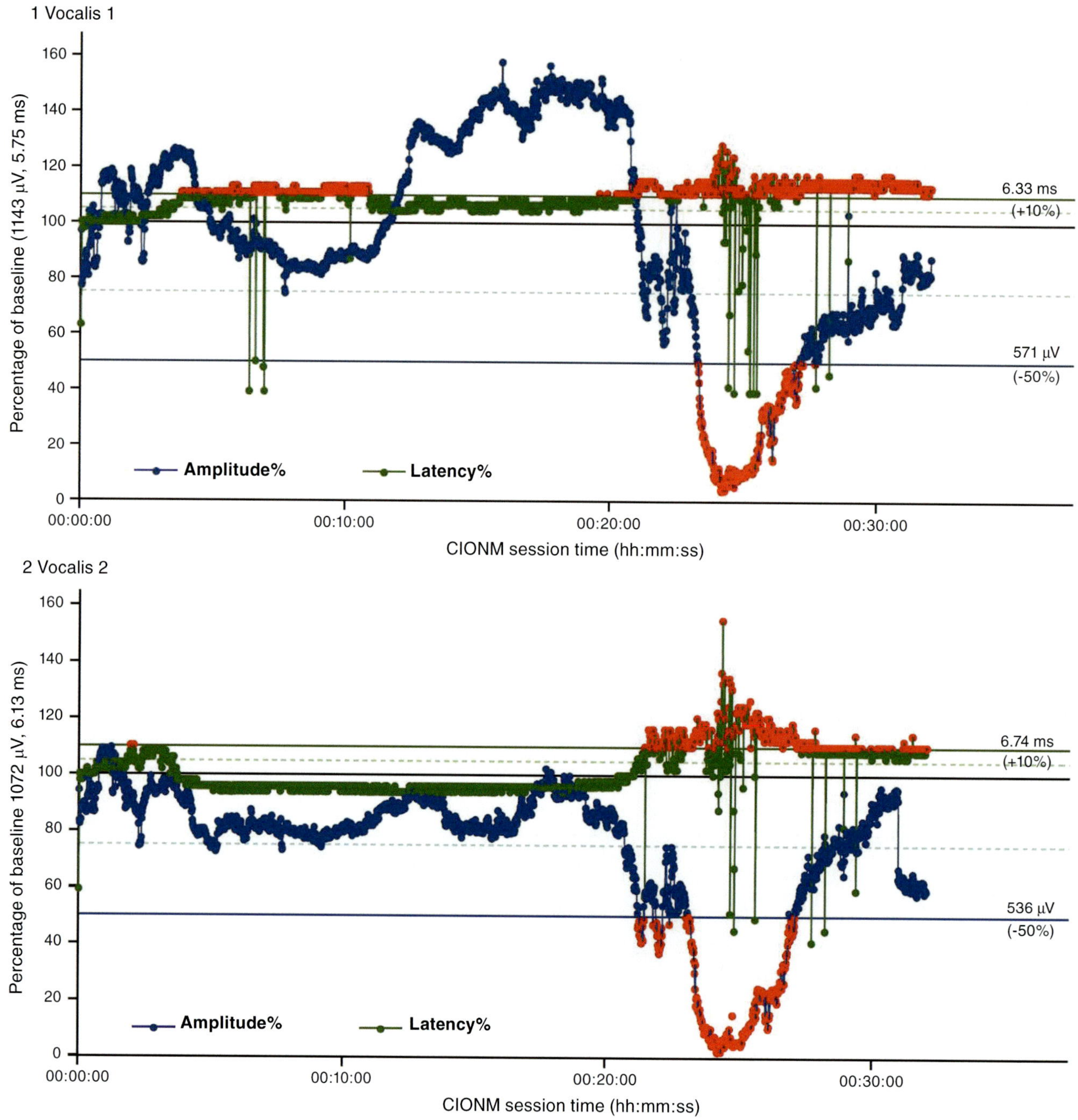


**Fig. 14.23** Transient global loss of signal (type 2) after traction on the left thyroid, after preceding combined event with progression of simultaneous amplitude decrease and latency increase, and intraoperative recovery of EMG signal with amplitude recovery >50% of baseline and normal postoperative vocal cord function

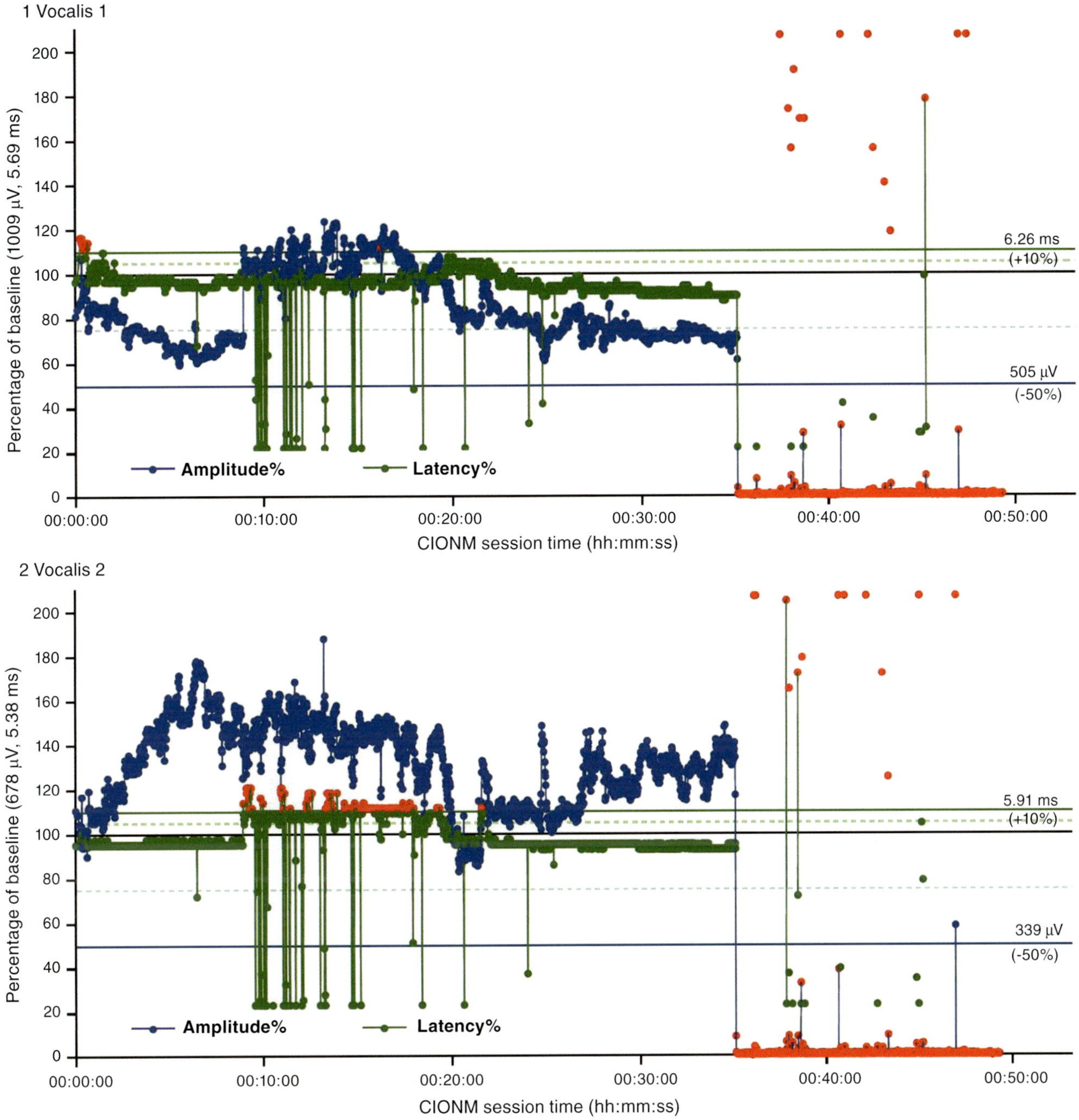


**Fig. 14.24** Definitive segmental loss of signal (type 1) after bipolar coagulation close to the recurrent laryngeal nerve on the left side, in which the nerve monitoring signal is lost all of a sudden with drop of amplitude, but without intraoperative recovery and 95 % risk for (transient) early postoperative vocal cord palsy

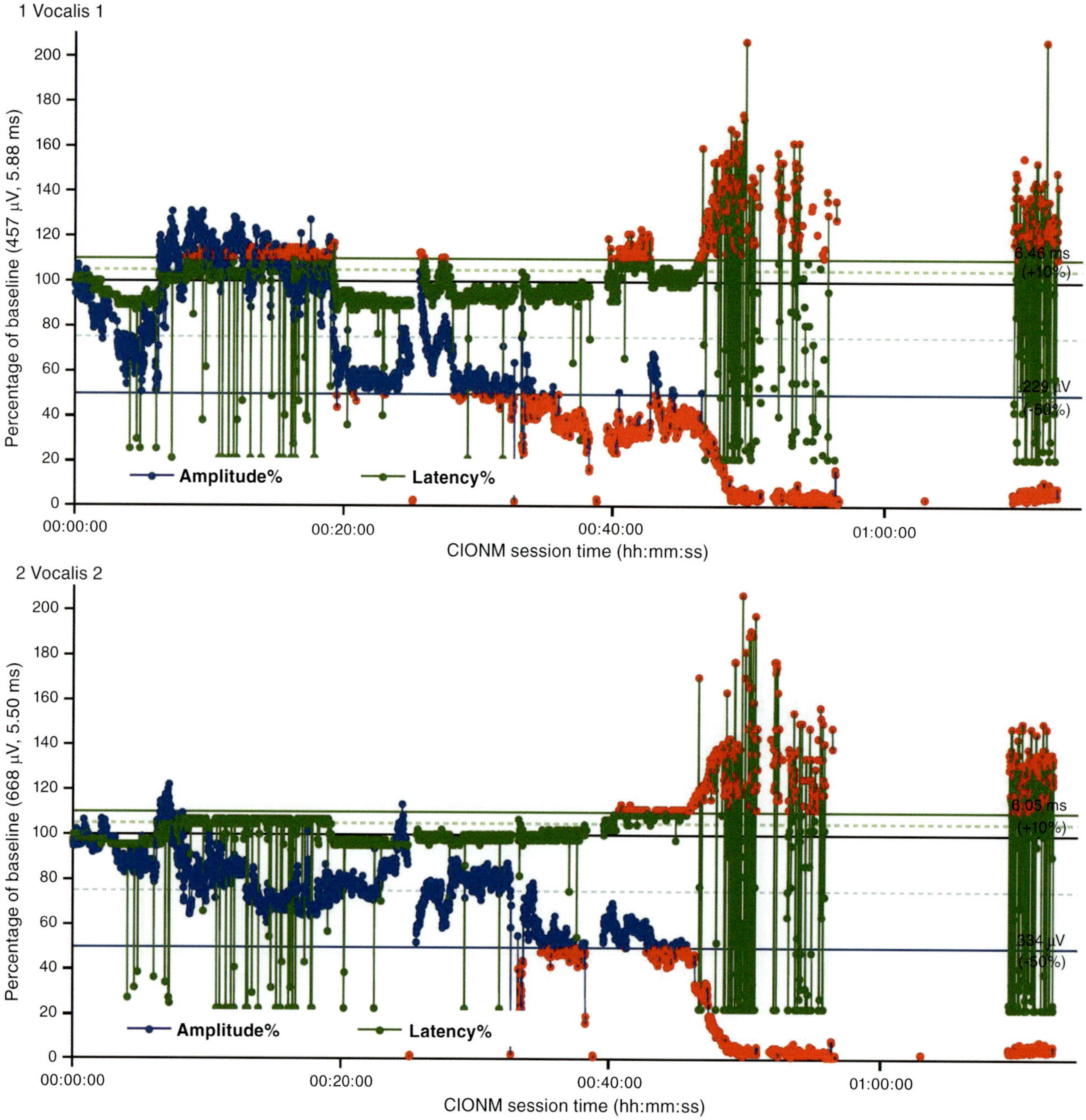


**Fig. 14.25** Definitive global loss of signal (type 2) after traction on the left thyroid, after preceding combined event with progression of simultaneous amplitude decrease and latency increase, but without intraoperative recovery and 70% risk for (transient) early postoperative vocal cord palsy

## References

1. Schneider R, Machens A, Randolph G, Kamani D, Lorenz K, Dralle H. Impact of continuous intraoperative vagus stimulation on intraoperative decision making in favor of or against bilateral surgery in benign goiter. Best Pract Res Clin Endocrinol Metab. 2019;33:101285.
2. Schneider R, Machens A, Sekulla C, Lorenz K, Weber F, Dralle H. Twenty-year experience of paediatric thyroid surgery using intraoperative nerve monitoring. Br J Surg. 2018;105:996–1005.
3. Schneider R, Machens A, Bucher M, Raspé C, Heinroth K, Dralle H. Continuous intraoperative monitoring of vagus and recurrent laryngeal nerve function in patients with advanced atrioventricular block. Langenbeck's Arch Surg. 2016;401:551–6.
4. Friedrich C, Ulmer C, Rieber F, Kern E, Kohler A, Schymik K, et al. Safety analysis of vagal nerve stimulation for continuous nerve monitoring during thyroid surgery. Laryngoscope. 2012;122:1979–87.
5. Schneider R, Randolph GW, Sekulla C, Phelan E, Thanh PN, Bucher M, et al. Continuous intraoperative vagus nerve stimulation for identification of imminent recurrent laryngeal nerve injury. Head Neck. 2013;35:1591–8.
6. Schneider R, Randolph G, Dionigi G, Barczynski M, Chiang FY, Wu CW, et al. Prediction of postoperative vocal fold function after intraoperative recovery of loss of signal. The International Neuromonitoring Study Group's PREC study. Laryngoscope. 2019;129:525–31.
7. Schneider R, Randolph GW, Dionigi G, Wu CW, Barczynski M, Chiang FY, et al. International neural monitoring study group guideline 2018 part I: staging bilateral thyroid surgery with monitoring loss of signal. Laryngoscope. 2018;128(Suppl 3):S1–S17.
8. Schneider R, Machens A, Sekulla C, Lorenz K, Elwerr M, Dralle H. Superiority of continuous over intermittent intraoperative nerve monitoring in preventing vocal cord palsy. Br J Surg. 2021;108:566–73.
9. Hsieh CY, Tan H, Huang HF, Huang TY, Wu CW, Chang PY, et al. Optimization of intraoperative neural monitoring of the recurrent laryngeal nerve in thyroid surgery. Medicina. 2022;58:495.
10. Randolph GW, Dralle H, Abdullah H, Barczynski M, Bellantone R, Brauckhoff M, et al. Electrophysiologic recurrent laryngeal nerve monitoring during thyroid and parathyroid surgery: international standards guideline statement. Laryngoscope. 2011;121:S1–S16.
11. Dionigi G, Chiang FY, Rausei S, Wu CW, Boni L, Lee KW, et al. Surgical anatomy and neurophysiology of the vagus nerve (VN) for standardised intraoperative neuromonitoring (IONM) of the inferior laryngeal nerve (ILN) during thyroidectomy. Langenbeck's Arch Surg. 2010;395:893–9.
12. Liddy W, Wu CW, Dionigi G, Donatini G, Giles Senyurek Y, Kamani D, et al. Varied recurrent laryngeal nerve course is associated with increased risk of nerve dysfunction during thyroidectomy: results of the surgical anatomy of the recurrent laryngeal nerve in thyroid surgery study, an International Multicenter Prospective Anatomic and Electrophysiologic Study of 1000 monitored nerves at risk from the International Neural Monitoring Study Group. Thyroid. 2021;31:1730–40.

# 15 Intraoperative Neuromonitoring of the RLNs During TOETVA Procedures

Özer Makay, Servet Celik, Gianlorenzo Dionigi, Francesco Frattini, and Antonella Pino

## Introduction

Many alternative approaches to the conventional open thyroid gland surgery have been developed, which are more likely to occur in women. One of these approaches is the "transoral endoscopic thyroidectomy with vestibular approach (TOETVA)." This remote-access procedure facilitates thyroid resection via small incisions on the inside of the lower lip, without a cutaneous scar (Fig. 15.1). Also called as "scarless" or "hidden-scar" thyroidectomy, this procedure is a suitable surgical option with proven safety and feasibility for a carefully selected patient population [1].

Besides thyroid and neck anatomy, it is of utmost importance to carry the knowledge of every detail regarding facial anatomy, especially the perioral and mentum region (Fig. 15.2). Static and dynamic actions during trocar insertion and port manipulations are involved with different anatomical structures that may be prone to injury. Nevertheless, dissection for thyroidectomy is carried out in the craniocaudal fashion. The surgeon is advised for the craniocaudal anatomical position of all anatomical structures (Fig. 15.3), concentrating especially on the entrance of the recurrent laryngeal nerve into the larynx (Fig. 15.4), the course of the recurrent laryngeal nerve and the parathyroid tissues [2].

The mental nerve is the sensory branch aroused from the inferior alveolar nerve (Fig. 15.5), which is separated from the mandibular branch of the trigeminal nerve (the cranial nerve V). If it is injured, it causes loss of sensation in the mucosal and cutaneous areas of the lower lip and chin. Patients may have difficulty in keeping food in their mouth and they may be able to bite their lower lips during chewing. Not only the root but also the distal branches of the mental nerve must be taken into consideration for safe surgery (Fig. 15.6) [3–5].

Ö. Makay (✉)
Department of General Surgery, Division of Endocrine Surgery, Ege University Hospital, Genel Cerrahi Kliniği, Izmir, Turkey

S. Celik
Department of Anatomy, Faculty of Medicine, Ege University, Izmir, Turkey
e-mail: servet.celik@ege.edu.tr

G. Dionigi · A. Pino
Division of Surgery, Istituto Auxologico Italiano IRCCS (Istituto di Ricovero e Cura a Carattere Scientifco), Milan, Italy
e-mail: gianlorenzo.dionigi@unimi.it

F. Frattini
Division of General and Bariatric Surgery, Istituto Auxologico Italiano, IRCCS, Milan, Italy
e-mail: f.frattini@auxologico.it


A. L. Shifrin et al. (eds.), *Atlas of Intraoperative Cranial Nerve Monitoring in Thyroid and Head and Neck Surgery*,
https://doi.org/10.1007/978-3-031-24613-5_15

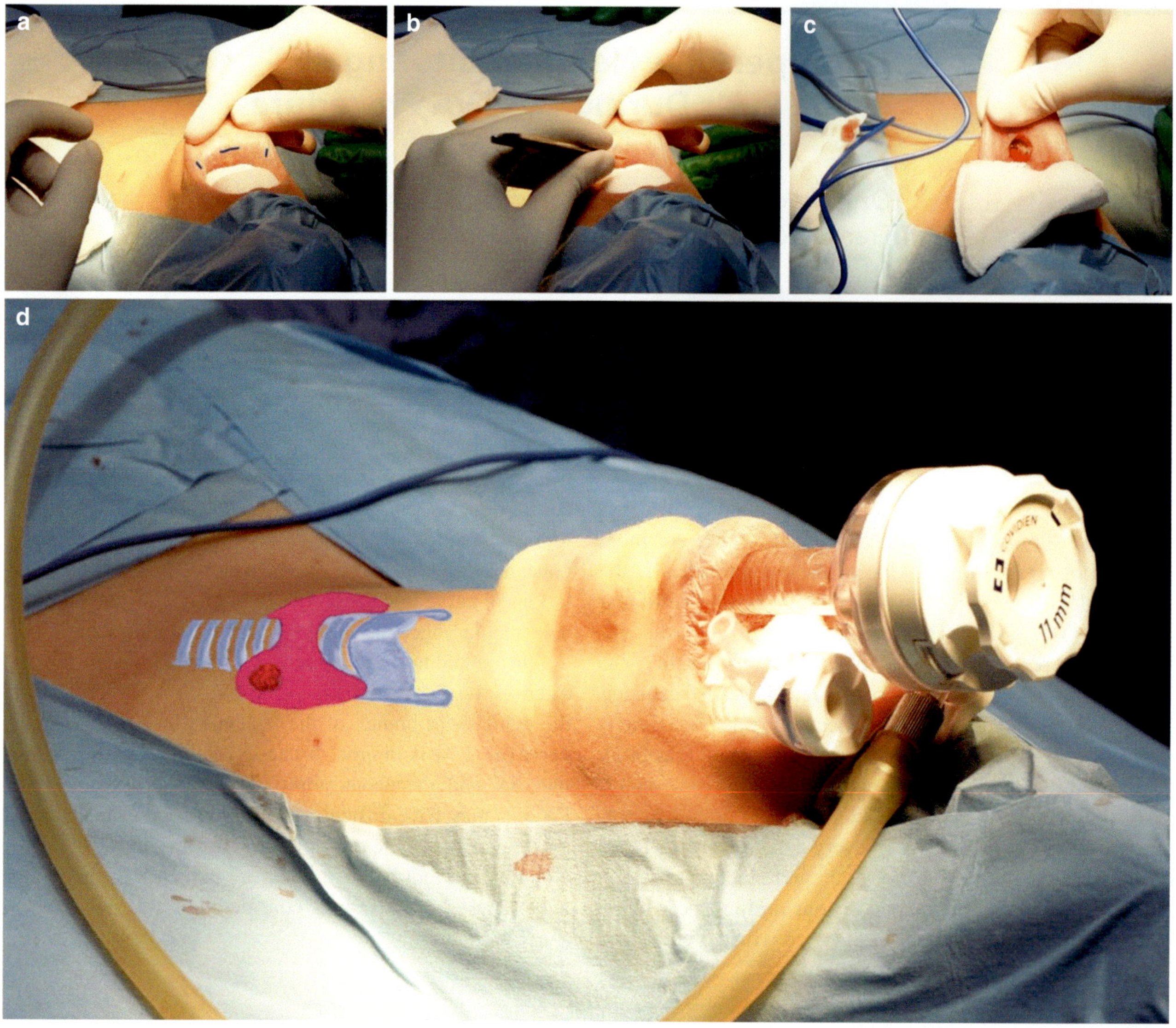

**Fig. 15.1** Initial steps of TOETVA. (**a**) Marking vestibular incisions of TOETVA; (**b**) executing median vestibular incision; (**c**) completing the median incision; (**d**) trocars of TOETVA inserted through the vestibular incisions

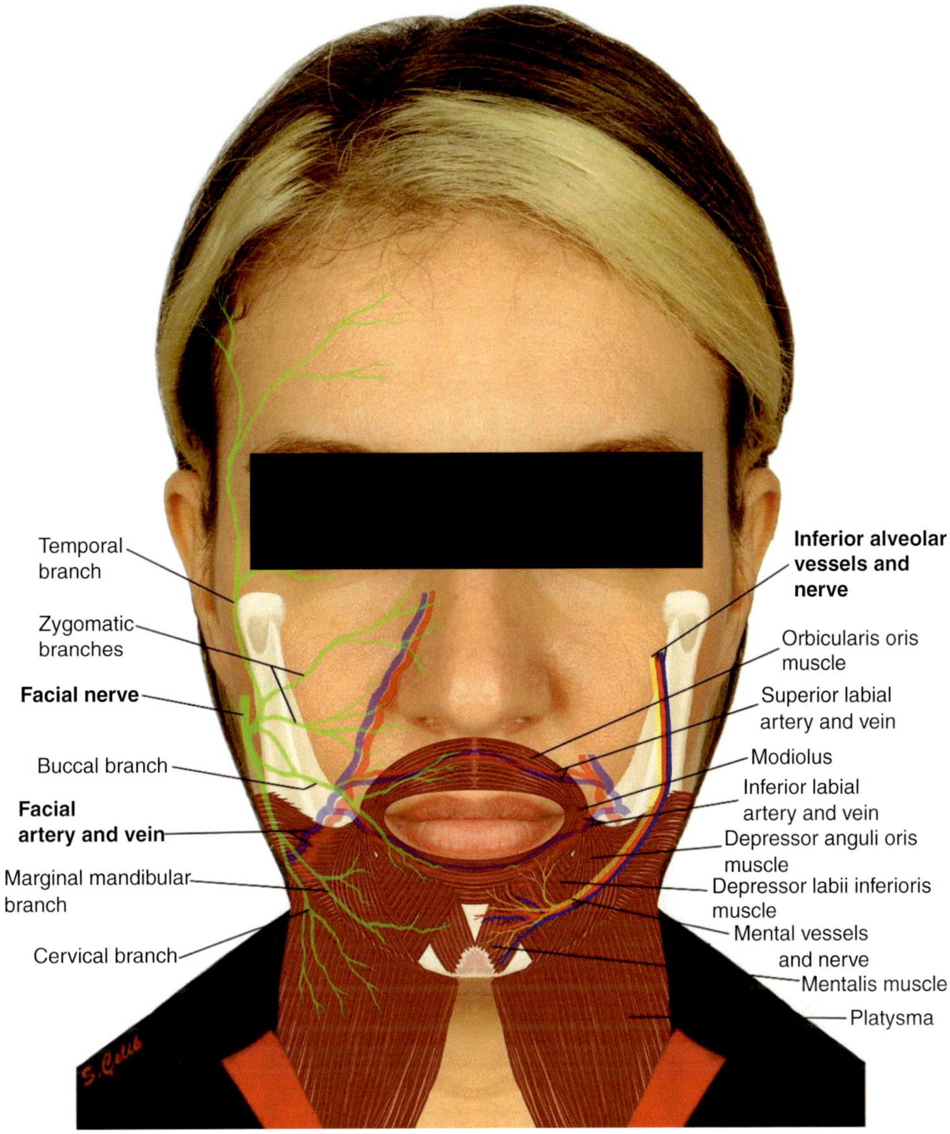


**Fig. 15.2** Facial, perioral, and mental anatomy related to TOETVA

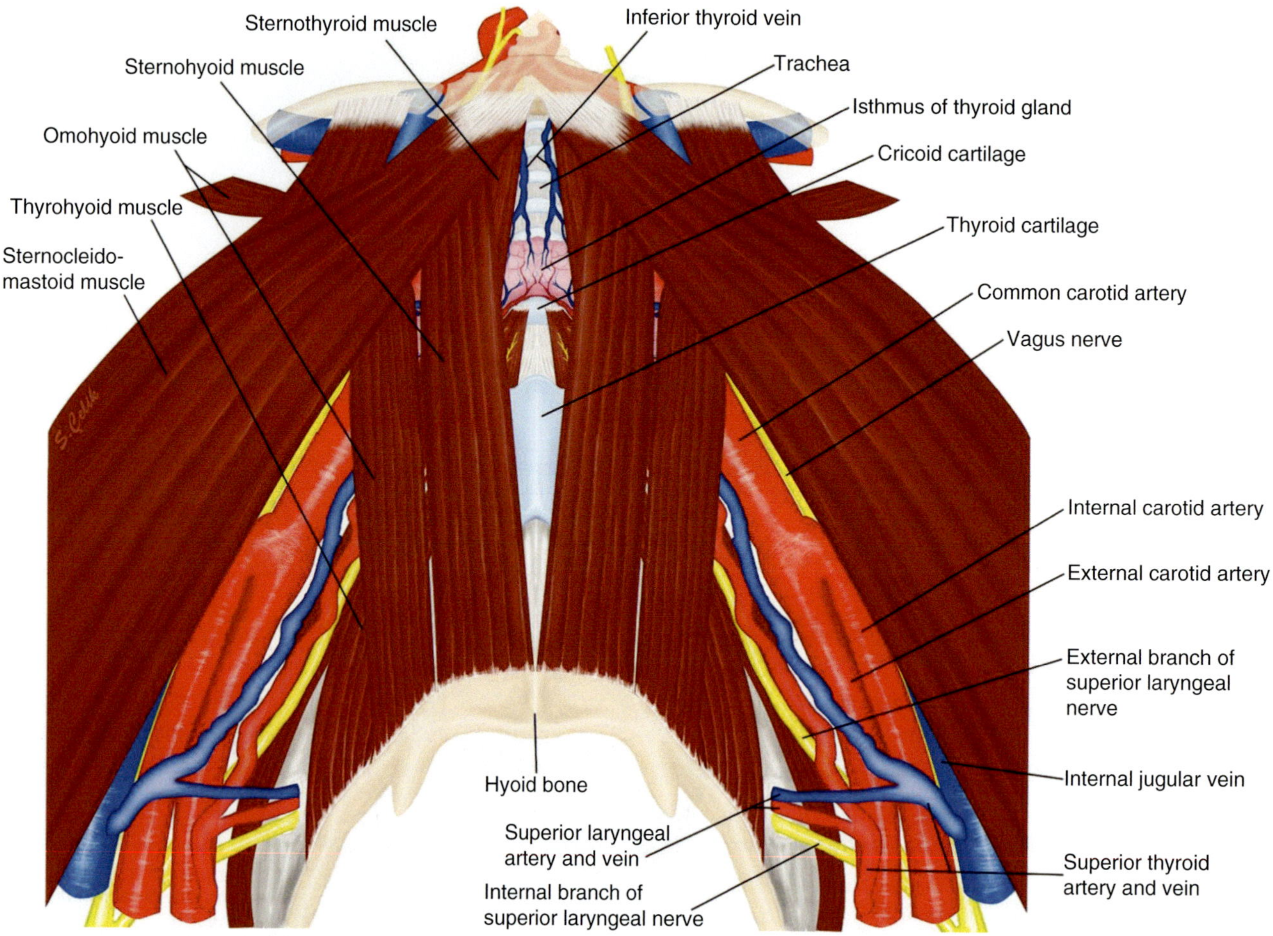


**Fig. 15.3** Craniocaudal position of neck anatomy required for TOETVA orientation

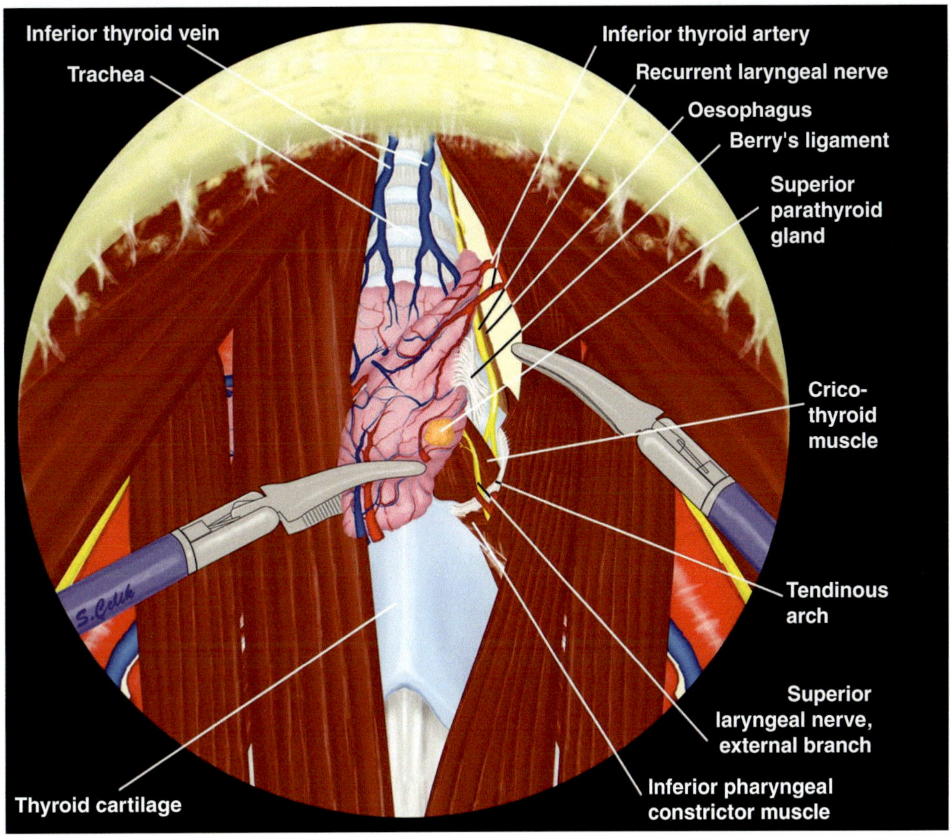


**Fig. 15.4** The recurrent laryngeal nerve in craniocaudal aspect

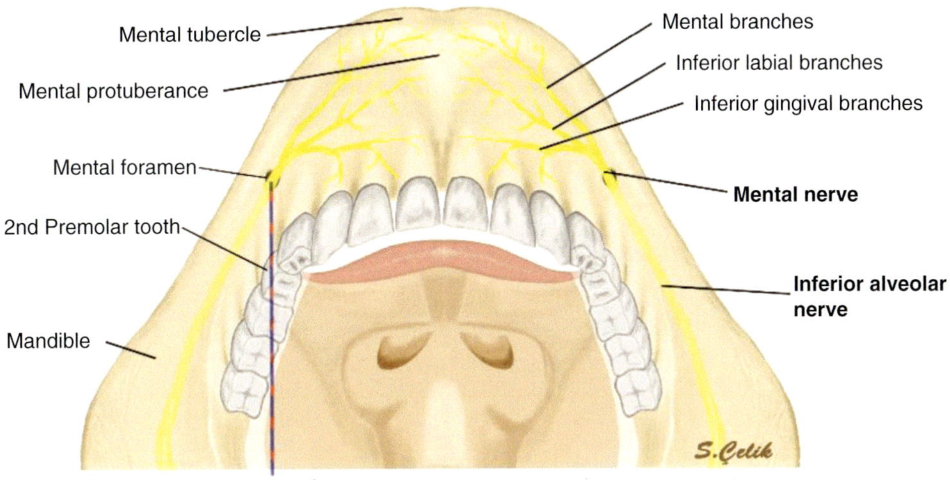


**Fig. 15.5** Course of the mental nerve and branches in craniocaudal aspect

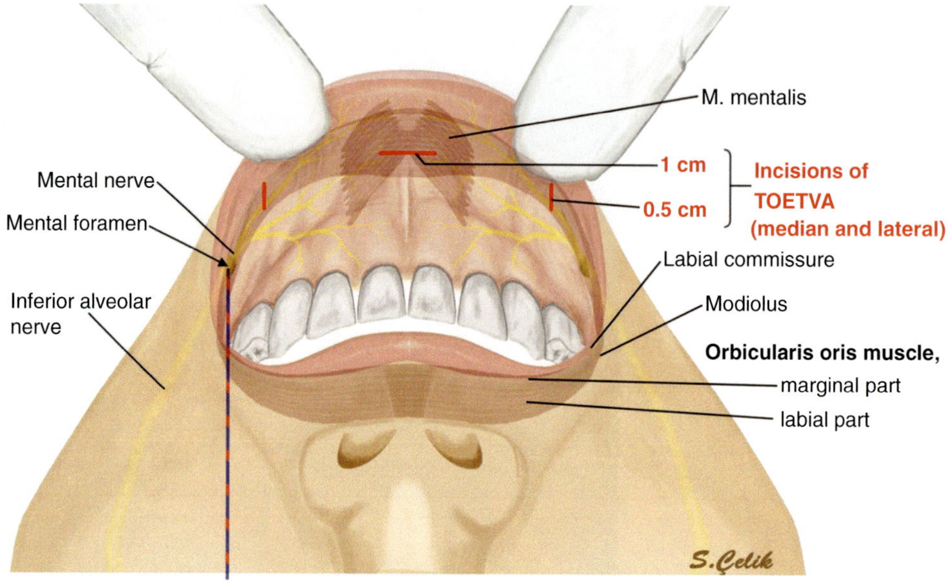


**Fig. 15.6** Relations of the mental nerve and branches concerning vestibular incisions of TOETVA

## The RLN Approach and Dissection in TOETVA

Both right and left RLNs were identified at the laryngeal entry point, which is the most consistent landmark for the RLN exposure in TOETVA. Other rational and anatomical references for nerve identification are the upper parathyroid glands (if they are in their usual location). The RLNs dissection is followed from cranial to caudal, with a top-down view. Early nerve exposure is guaranteed by (a) ligation of the upper thyroid vessels, (b) raising of the upper pole of the thyroid, (c) identification of the superior ipsilateral parathyroid gland. Landmark for nerve identification and initial dissection is limited to the laryngeal entry point and superior parathyroid gland.

After the superior pole has been lifted, the dissection continues with separating the superior thyroidal vessels with energy device. During the course of lateral dissection, superior parathyroid glands are identified and protected. In this process, the RLN is made sure to be identified at the entry point. The RLN stimulation is achieved by a long probe, percutaneously placed monopolar probe, and adapted Maryland dissector connected to the IONM system (Fig. 15.7). IONM is useful for identifying and confirming the RLN in the transoral approach and facilitates mapping the RLN course and dissecting the nerve.

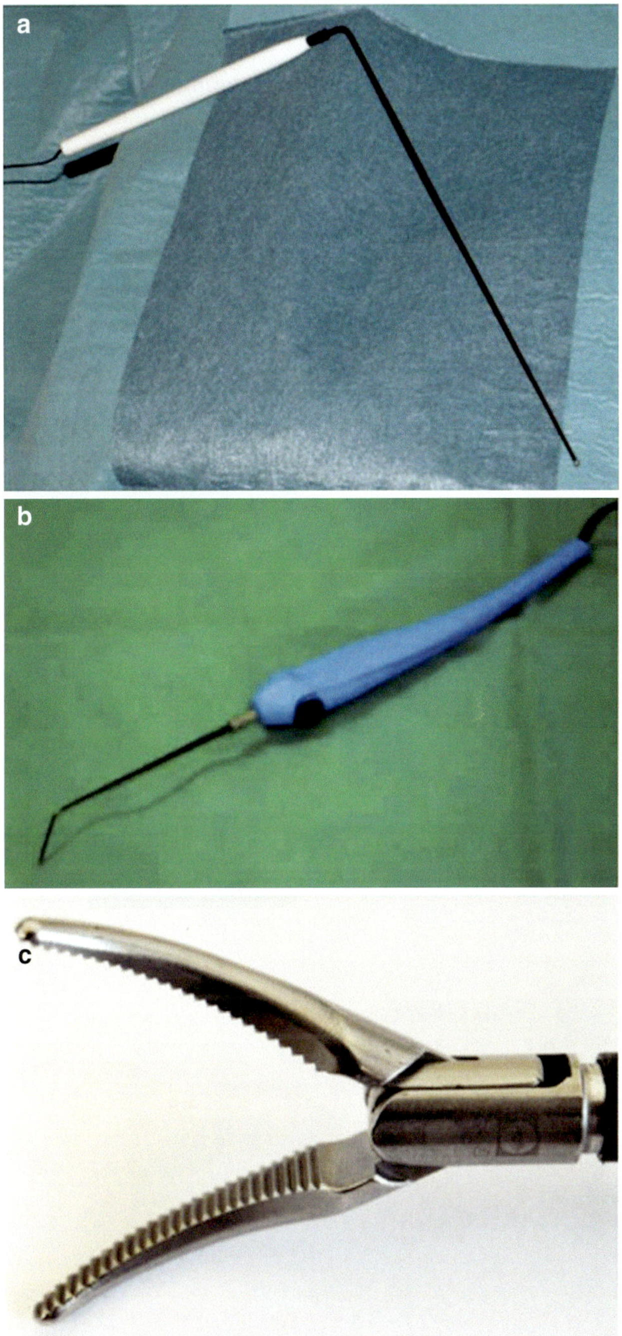


**Fig. 15.7** Stimulating probes with three different tools (*from* Zhang et al. [6]; *with permission*)

## The RLN Injury During TOETVA 2

Overall incidence of the RLN injury during TOETVA is 3.1–4.3%. Temporary and permanent RLN injury rates are similar to that of open thyroidectomy.

Although IONM is routinely used for the RLN identification, the RLN palsy still occurs. Nearly 80% of the lesions are located at the distal 1 cm of the course of the RLN. The surgeons may face two types of injury: Type 1 (segmental) and Type 2 (diffuse) RLN injuries. With LOS, two issues should be considered: (I) identification of the site of lesion—that is, neural injury point mapping and (II) consideration of optimal contralateral surgery timing. The "LOS troubleshooting algorithm" should be applied systematically (Fig. 15.8).

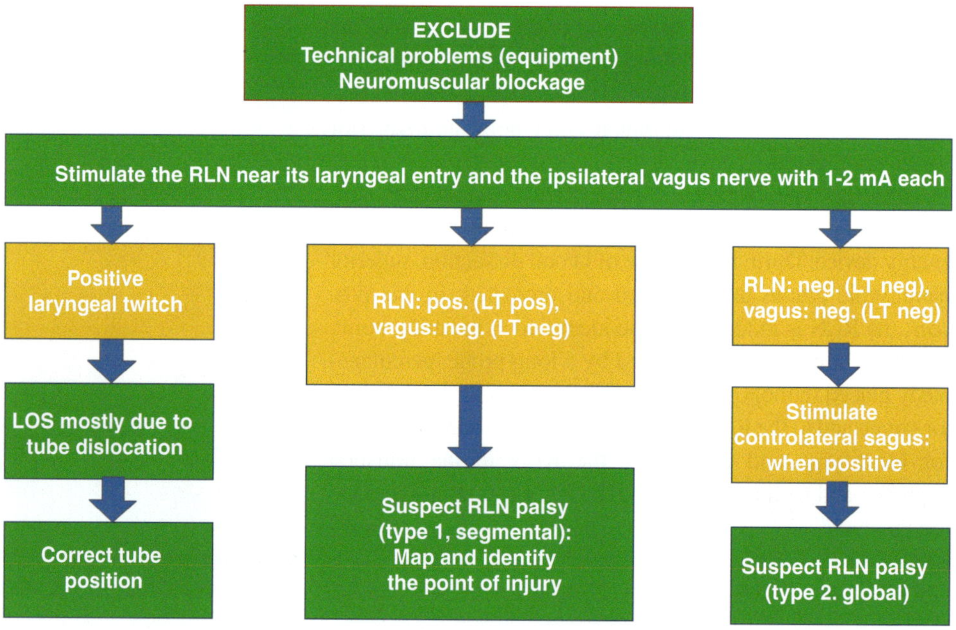


**Fig. 15.8** Troubleshooting algorithm after LOS during TOETVA (*from* Zhang et al. [6]; *with permission*)

## The EBSLN Approach and Dissection in TOETVA

The EBSLN is in closed anatomical proximity to the superior thyroid vessels and can be easily injured when the vessels of the superior thyroid are separated close to the gland. The identification of the EBSLN is challenging from the perspective of TOETVA surgery in a cephalic to caudal manner. In addition, in endoscopic surgery the thermal damage by the ultrasonic device used in thyroid dissection may cause injury to the EBSLN.

Several studies assessed that IONM was a more effective method than traditional visualization in localizing the EBSLN.

After transection of sternothyroid muscle from the thyroid lobe EBSLN should be exposed in the avascular space between the larynx medially and the superior pole laterally. The use of IONM to detect the course of the EBSLN is documented to be the best option to avoid injury to the EBSLN during TOETVA. The stimulation of the EBSLN at 1.0 mA is assessed by cricothyroid muscle twitch and by electromyographic signal (Fig. 15.9).

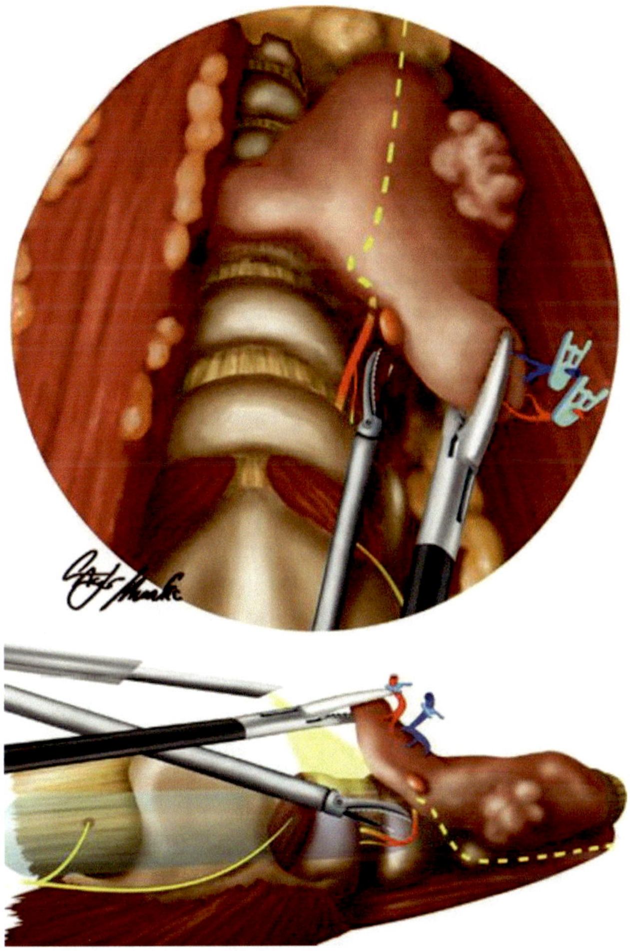

**Fig. 15.9** The EBSLN identification in cephalic to caudal manner (*from* Zhang et al. [7]; *with permission*)

## IONM Key Steps in TOETVA

Monitored TOETVA is performed according to standards of equipment setup, induction and maintenance anesthesia, correct tube positioning verification tests, EMG definitions described by the INMSG Guidelines, as usually described in open thyroidectomy. Several reports described the techniques for the recurrent laryngeal nerve (RNL) monitoring in TOETVA. However, many techniques described and used in open procedures are not exploitable in TOETVA. Thus, for safety, utility, simplicity, systems rely on endotracheal tube-based surface electrodes for TOETVA.

TOETVA is performed under general anesthesia with naso- or orotracheal intubation. The medium long-acting muscle relaxant (Rocuronium) should be administered as a low dose (0.3 mg/kg). The EMG endotracheal tube is fixed at the right corner of the mouth and equipment for anesthesia is set up on the same side of the patient. The endotracheal tube tape is fixed on the upper lip, not on the lower as it is involved during the early stages of dissection.

The rationale of IONM, used before performing any surgical maneuver during TOETVA, is to explore the growing direction of the RLN, identify the RLN reliably, and verify the functional integrity of the RLN. The vagal nerve was routinely tested (V1) with a current of 3 mA to ensure that the monitoring system be functional. With the guidance of IONM using stimulation level of 3 mA, the localization of the RLN was evaluated, and gentle blunt dissection was performed to explore the RLN at its cervical entry point. The RLN was identified relying on laryngeal electromyography (EMG) responses with the stimulation level of 1 mA. The EMG signal of R1 was recorded by a current of 1 mA after exposure of the RLN. After the whole operation, signals of the RLN and the vagal nerve were obtained by stimulation as R2 and V2, respectively. The different IONM stimulation levels were chosen according to the operative purpose; if the surgeon needs to evaluate the location of the RLN, a high level (3 mA or more) would be appropriate, while if the purpose was to identify the RLN or confirm its integrity, a low level (1 mA) would be better. Thyroid dissection was implemented by tracing the growing direction of the RLN carefully. During the procedure, the functional scalpel or energy-based device used should be kept away from the RLN all the time, preventing thermal damage to the nerves. The aim of preventing the RLN injury at its entry point can be easily achieved due to the clear vision of "up to down" (Fig. 15.10). After the procedure of dissecting the thyroid capsule away from the RLN, the Berry's ligament was identified and divided. During this procedure, the device can be rotated vertically to obtain a better operative vision. In addition, the inferior parathyroid gland with its vascular pedicle is also identified and could be preserved carefully. Then after the thyroid lobe was lifted medially with a grasp for-

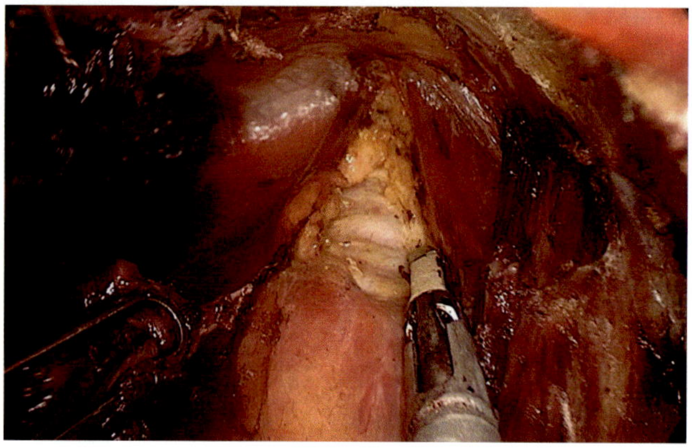

**Fig. 15.10** Intraoperative endoscopic craniocaudal view after dissection of the thyroid isthmus for identification of laryngeal nerve the RLN

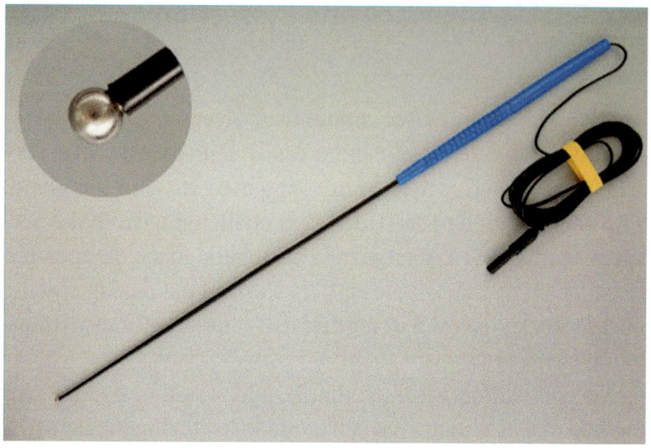

**Fig. 15.11** Long stimulation probe with round tip

ceps, the lower pole was identified and divided from perithyroidal tissues. During the upper pole dissection, before any surgical maneuver, also the external branch of superior laryngeal nerve (EBSLN) is stimulated cranially and caudally to the superior vascular peduncle, with the objective of ensuring the preservation and its functional integrity. The evocated response must be considered positive when it produces the contraction or twitch of the cricothyroid muscle.

To apply intermitted intraoperative neuromonitoring (IONM) of the recurrent laryngeal nerve (RLN) in transoral endoscopic thyroidectomy vestibular approach, several varieties of electrodes have been proposed as percutaneously placed hand-stimulating probe commonly used in open surgery, long probes placed through the trocar, adapting endoscopic Maryland dissecting instruments to the IONM system, and flexible electrode wires. Each mode of application has advantages and disadvantages.

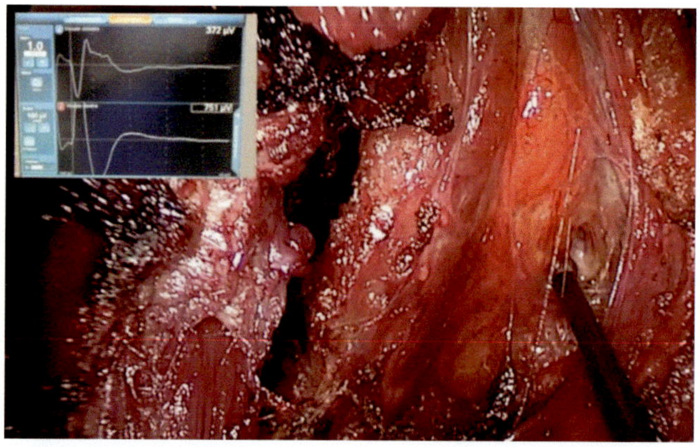

**Fig. 15.12** Identification and monitoring of the RLN and EBSLN (the figure shows the intraoperative view of a lobe already mobilized medially with the lower and upper poles in evidence with the tip of the probe in direct contact with the nerve)

## IONM Procedure with Long Stimulating Probe

With a long stimulating probe, through the trocar, stimulation of both V1 and V2 was achieved without carotid sheath dissection by simply and gently applying probe on the carotid sheath with 2–3 mA stimulation intensity. Monitored TOETVA with the long stimulating probe is feasible and safe (Fig. 15.11). There were no instances of IONM equipment interference with the other endoscopic instruments. The first advantage is that IONM facilitates the RLN and the SLN identification (Fig. 15.12). Second, it enables testing of the RLN and the SLN function. Third, it enables corrective action at three stages of surgery: (I) during blunt dissection; (II) during use of energy-based devices, and (III) during thyroid gland retraction. Notably, retraction of thyroid gland by grasp forceps or by forceps can cause excessive traction and subsequent functional damage of the RLN. Fourth, it enables evaluation of the RLN function by vagal nerve stimulation on one side before proceeding to the contralateral lobe. This advantage is particularly important for bilaterally approaches. The fifth advantage is that, for novice surgeons, IONM increases confidence in performing TOETVA procedures. However, skilled surgeons can also use IONM to explore new applications of TOETVA.

Summing up, the advantages of using the long stimulating probe are: (a) achievement of the vagal nerve (V1, V2), the recurrent laryngeal nerve (R1, R2), and the superior laryngeal nerve (S1, S2) determinations; (b) no additional neck skin incisions; (c) precise contact with nerve structure and thus, use of lower intensity stimulation; (d) versatility (i.e., bilateral use, both lobes dissection, both laryngeal nerves mapping, any port insertion); (e) atraumatic (i.e., ball tip); (f) tip is flexible, can be adjusted during procedure to reach narrow areas of dissection; (g) the long stimulating probe is FDA approved. Possible limits are: (a) availability of the long probe in the operating room and additional cost related; (b) changing instrument; (c) some loss of $CO_2$ insufflation from port; (d) currently the long stimulating probe is not available in the incrementing probe/remote control mode of application; (e) disposable.

## IONM Guidance with Percutaneous Stimulating Probe

A disposable monopolar ball-tipped stimulating probe (1.0 mm) with a 10-cm handle and a 9-cm shaft is used for nerve stimulation through a percutaneous approach. A 0.5-cm circle was drawn on the side of the dominant thyroid lesion, with its midpoint at the intersection of a line 2 cm lateral to the anterior median line and a line 2 cm above the line connecting the bilateral clavicular heads (Fig. 15.13). After ensuring that there are no major vessels within the puncture site in this circle, the skin is pierced with an 18-gage hypodermic needle. After the needle was withdrawn, the probe was carefully inserted through the needle channel (Fig. 15.14). The tool is usually guided by the first assistant. During dissection from the junction of the inferior thyroid artery and the recurrent laryngeal nerve to the larynx, the probe tip is gently held on the vagal nerve to allow its neuromonitoring, also in APS mode.

As specified for the stimulation with the long probe, the percutaneous technique also brings advantages and disadvantages. The advantages of using percutaneous stimulating probe are: (a) availability (i.e., same instrument open procedure); (b) tip flexibility; (c) atraumatic ball tip; (d) no need to use ports. Possible limits are: (a) additional step/procedure (i.e., further skin neck incision); (b) two more skin incisions for bilateral procedure; (c) possible $CO_2$ insufflation leak; (d) tip wearing; (e) hindrance when held in place; (f) disposable.

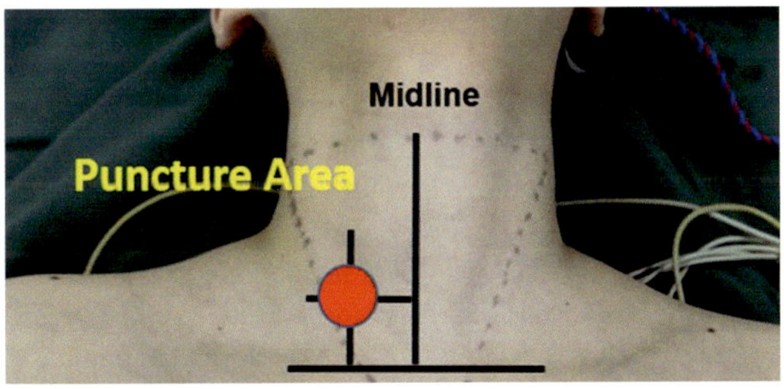


**Fig. 15.13** Puncture point for nerve-monitoring probe entry (the figure shows the anatomical drawing of the neck with a precise indication of where to puncture for the insertion of the probe, drawing on the neck the intersection of two lines that mark the puncture area, as indicated in the main text) (*from* Zhang et al. [8]; Creative Commons Attribution License [CC BY 4.0]; https://creativecommons.org/licenses/by/4.0/)

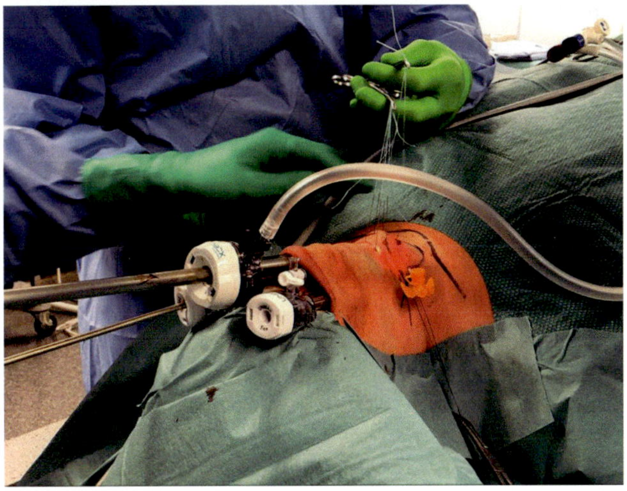

**Fig. 15.14** Positioning of probe (the figure indicates the operating field with the probe passing through the skin tissues through the cannula of the 18-gage needle with which the puncture was performed before)

## IONM Operative Strategy with Dissecting and Stimulating Instruments

Intraoperative neuromonitoring (IONM) has been introduced to facilitate identification and verify functional integrity of the RLN in thyroid surgery. The system is based on a dedicated endotracheal tube with two paired wires (less than 1 mm in diameter) incorporated into the wall of the endotracheal tube and exposed 30 mm at the glottis level for optimal bilateral vocal cord mucosa contact. The tube is interfaced with an EMG monitor through a connector box.

The system allows evoked surface EMG monitoring of the left and right thyroarytenoid muscles during stimulation of the RLN and the vagus nerve in monitored thyroid and parathyroid surgery. In this way the thyroid surgeon can hear and see the recorded EMG activity of both vocal cords.

Care must be taken in positioning the electrode accurately as the adjustment of the head and neck after intubation can change the relative position of the tube and hence the electrodes. By using IONM, the laryngeal nerves are identified, mapped, stimulated, and monitored in the surgical field by the application of a sterile, single use, pulse-generated monopolar stimulator probe.

Monitored TOETVA is performed according to standards of equipment setup, induction and maintenance anesthesia, correct tube positioning verification tests, EMG (electromyography) definitions described by the International Neural Monitoring Study Group (INMSG) Guidelines. Endotracheal tube-based surface electrodes for monitored TOETVA are preferred because of safety and simplicity of this system.

The standardization of an IONM technique, first described by Chang, is composed of four steps also in TOETVA

**Table 15.1** Standard algorithm for IONM technique

| | | |
|---|---|---|
| (I) | V1 | Test the vagus nerve before identification of the RLN |
| (II) | R1 | The RLN stimulation when it is identified at the tracheoesophageal groove |
| (III) | R2 | The RLN stimulation after it is completely dissected from the Berry's ligament |
| (IV) | V2 | Test the vagus nerve after complete hemostasis |

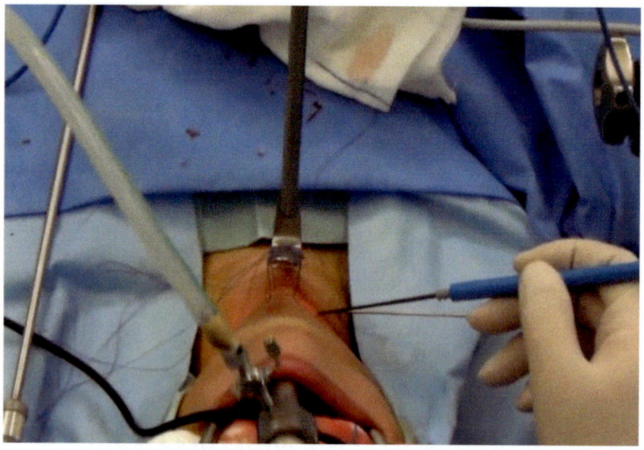

**Fig. 15.15** External image of stimulation with long probe

(Table 15.1). Early nerve exposure is guaranteed by (a) ligation of upper thyroid vessels, (b) raising of the upper pole of the thyroid, (c) identification of the superior ipsilateral parathyroid gland.

Landmark for nerve identification and initial dissection is limited to the laryngeal entry point and superior parathyroid gland. The RLN stimulation is achieved by a long probe, percutaneously placed monopolar probe, and adapted Maryland dissector connected to the IONM system (Fig. 15.15).

Platysma is raised from the level of mandible to the level of sternum and then laterally to sternocleidomastoid muscles under endoscopic screening. There is thyroid cartilage located in the upper margin of the flap, while lower margin is the sternal notch and lateral margins are the medial aspect of the sternocleidomastoid muscle. It is recommended that the dissection be proceeded down to the level of the thyroid cartilage notch and also median raphe of the strap be specified and divided in order to expose the thyroid gland. V1 response should be obtained before starting the thyroid tissue dissection.

The thyroid is split in the isthmus and the posterior surface of the isthmus is separated from the trachea to the ligament of Berry under craniocaudal view. We first lift the superior pole and following this continue with separating the superior thyroidal vessels with energy device.

During the course of lateral dissection, superior parathyroid glands are identified and protected. In this process, the RLN is made sure to be identified at the entry point. Then the gland is medially pulled back further, which would enable a capsular dissection. We continue the dissection by dissecting the ligament of Berry and the specimen obtained is taken through the camera port.

## Advanced Monitoring with C-IONM

The continuous IONM (C-IONM) enables early detection and warning of a change in the RLN function. A baseline of nerve function through the automatic periodic stimulation (APS) is obtained, and subsequent EMG responses are monitored and charted in real time to provide feedback. Unlike intermittent IONM, continuous IONM allows to prevent the recurrent laryngeal nerve injury.

APS is a biocompatible, soft-rubber, monopolar electrode. The APS electrode is available in two sizes: 2 mm and 3 mm, with some ability to adapt to any VN size and increased diameter avoiding squeezing and compression trauma to the nerve itself.

Considering the increase in VN size during dissection and surgery for local edema and in order to avoid compression-related injuries, an important feature of C-IONM electrode must be an atraumatic design and, of note, its adaptability over time during the surgical intervention.

The APS accessory is wet before to facilitate its sliding into the left 5-mm port. Also, the outer black clip is carefully removed. The APS electrode is placed through the left 5-mm port. The port is then removed by sliding the wire inside until the end and then restored. Therefore, the wire of the APS remains between the port and the vestibule. In this way, there is no interference with the introduction of the endoscopic instruments in the port.

The APS is positioned gently on the VN after opening the carotid sheet by a 2-cm pouch. Careful 360° dissection of the VN with Maryland forceps is required. To prevent VN thermal injuries, energy-based devices were avoided (Figs. 15.16 and 15.17).

As for the I-IONM, its use is much more challenging in TOETVA. C-IONM was feasible in TOETVA in porcine models, but simplification of electrode design and applica-

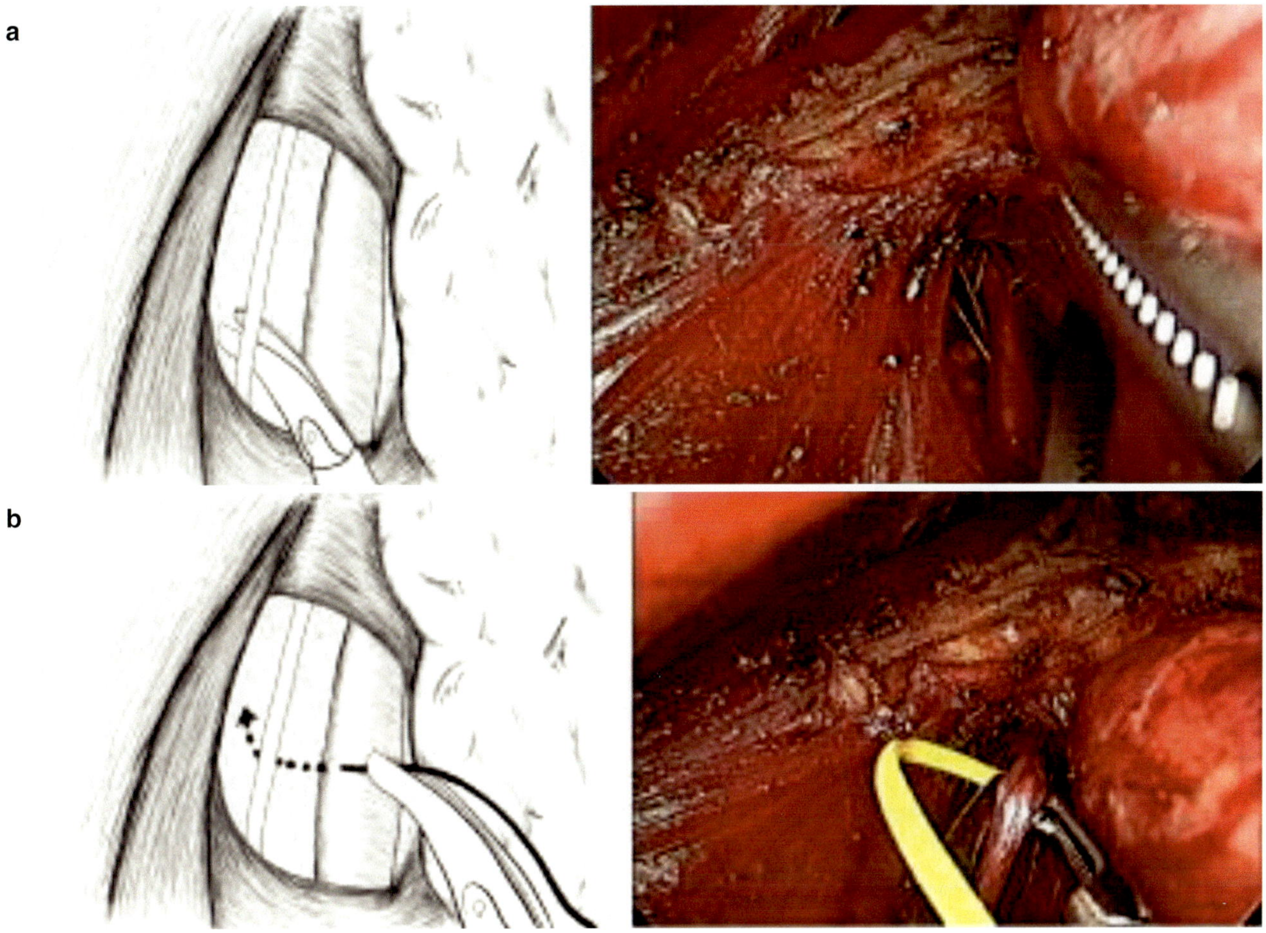

**Fig. 15.16** An endoscopic image focusing on dissection and identification of the vagus nerve. (**a**) Initial step of preparation of the vagus nerve. (**b**) Course of the vagus probe (*from* Chen et al. [9]; *with permission*)

tion is needed. Few case- series of c-IONM application in TOETVA in humans have been reported. These limited evidences assessed that the use of C-IONM is reliable and safe during transoral endoscopic thyroidectomies and may help in the early detection of adverse electromyographic mutations, thus preventing the RLN injury. This procedure can be challenging endoscopically, time-consuming, or even harmful to the nerve and vessels while positioning the accessory and at removal of the electrode. Furthermore, C-IONM accessory should be versatile because the position of the vagus nerve in relation to the common carotid artery and the internal jugular vein in humans is very changeable. In relation to the features of C-IONM electrodes available currently for thyroid surgery, none of these seems to be easy to apply in TOETVA.

Continuous neural stimulation was performed using the delta electrode device. The stimulation was set at 0.7 mA every 1 s. This enabled the ongoing assessment of stimulation waveform amplitude and latency EMG of the vocalis muscle was checked, and the alarm was set to activate when the EMG amplitude was decreased by 50% and latency was prolonged by 10%.

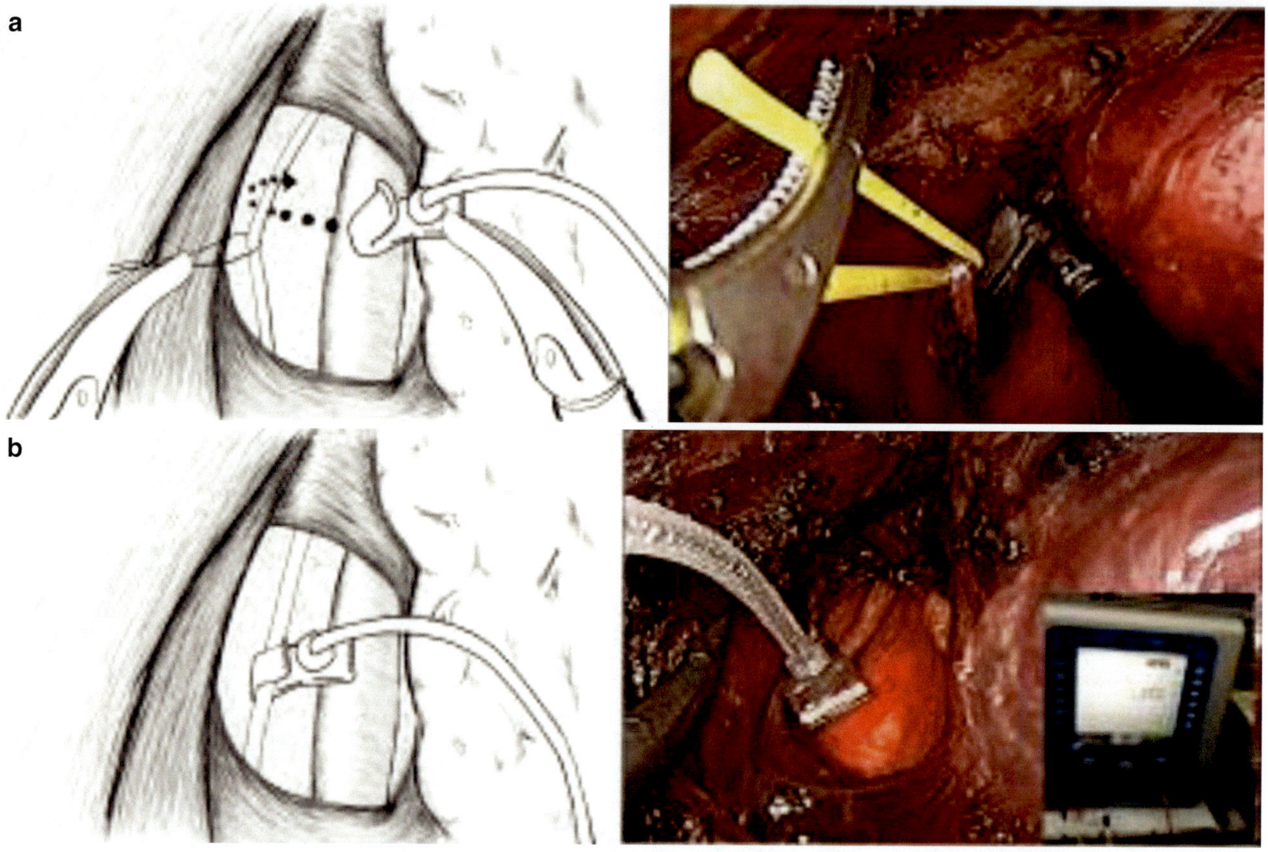


**Fig. 15.17** The picture represents an endoscopic view of the positioning of the delta electrode around the vagus nerve for continuous stimulation. (**a**) Management how to put the delta electrode. (**b**) Final positioning of the delta electrode (*from* Chen et al. [9]; *with permission*)

## IONM Limits in TOETVA

Significant limits of intraoperative neuromonitoring in transoral surgery are determined by:

(a) inability to appreciate the laryngeal twitch by digital palpation (and endoscopic vision),
(b) difficulty in stimulating the ipsilateral and contralateral vagus nerve without further surgical dissection and prolonged operative time,
(c) difficulty in the endotracheal tube position verification, and
(d) limited operative area for IONM probe (Fig. 15.18).

We suggest using increased current (3–10 mA) to facilitate mapping over the carotid sheath for VN stimulation. Short duration of high-current stimulus (3–10 mA) can be applied to facilitate indirect VN mapping/stimulation over the lateral neck region.

Most false LOS is due to EMG tube up displacement (upwards) because the chin/neck is more flexed ("sniff position") than extended during TOETVA. The overall prevalence of EMG tube displacement in TOETVA is 15%. For EMG tube displacement, because oral/nasal area is included in the aseptic field, it is less possible to re-check by the laryngoscope or fiberscope.

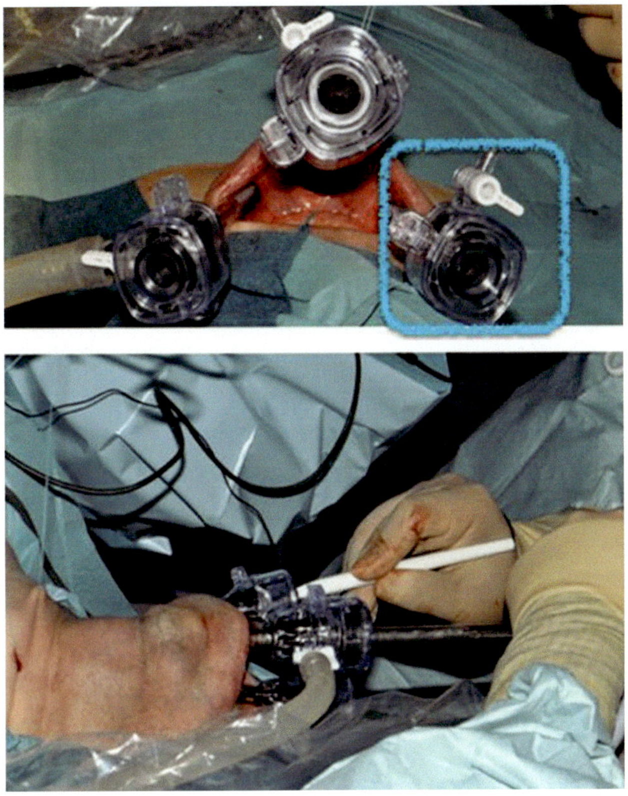

**Fig. 15.18** Significant limits of intraoperative neuromonitoring in transoral surgery are determined by the limited operative area for IONM probe (*from* Zhang et al. [6]; *with permission*)

## References


1. Anuwong A. Transoral endoscopic thyroidectomy vestibular approach: a series of the first 60 human cases. World J Surg. 2016;40:491–7.
2. Makay O, Dionigi G, Celik S. İzsiz Tiroidektomi Vestibüler Yaklaşim ile Transoral Endoskopik Tiroidektomi TOETVA Atlası. 1st ed. İstanbul: İstanbul Tıp Kitabevleri; 2018.
3. Celik S, Makay O, Yoruk MD, Kocer IB, Ozdemir M, Kilic KD, Tomruk C, Bilge O, Uyanikgil Y, Dionigi G. A surgical and anatomo-histological study on transoral endoscopic thyroidectomy vestibular approach (TOETVA). Surg Endosc. 2020;34:1088–102.
4. Zhang D, Fu Y, Dionigi G, Pontin A, Caruso E, Antonella P, Sun H. Human cadaveric model for studying the preservation of mental nerve during transoral endoscopic thyroidectomy. Surg Radiol Anat. 2020;42:55–62.
5. Zhang D, Famá F, Caruso E, Pinto G, Pontin A, Pino A, Mandolfino T, Gagliano E, Siniscalchi EN, De Ponte FS, Sun H, Dionigi G. How to avoid and manage mental nerve injury in transoral thyroidectomy. How to avoid and manage mental nerve injury in transoral thyroidectomy. Surg Technol Int. 2019;35:101–6.
6. Zhang D, Mazzeo C, Dionigi G, et al. Nerve monitoring for transoral thyroid surgery: why, how, and what to expect. Curr Otorhinolaryngol Rep. 2019;7:225–31. https://doi.org/10.1007/s40136-019-00251-z.
7. Zhang D, Sun H, Tufano R, Caruso E, Dionigi G, Kim HY. Recurrent laryngeal nerve management in transoral endoscopic thyroidectomy. Oral Oncol. 2020;108:104755. https://doi.org/10.1016/j.oraloncology.2020.104755. Epub 2020 Jun 8.
8. Zhang D, Wang C, Wang T, Du R, Li K, Yang M, Xue G, Dionigi G, Sun H. Clinical experience of use of percutaneous continuous nerve monitoring in robotic bilateral axillo-breast thyroid surgery. Front Endocrinol. 2022;12:817026. https://doi.org/10.3389/fendo.2021.817026.
9. Chen HK, Chen CL, Wen KS, et al. Application of transoral continuous intraoperative neuromonitoring in natural orifice transluminal endoscopic surgery for thyroid disease: a preliminary study. Surg Endosc. 2018;32:517–25. https://doi.org/10.1007/s00464-017-5656-0.

# Index





A. L. Shifrin et al. (eds.), *Atlas of Intraoperative Cranial Nerve Monitoring in Thyroid and Head and Neck Surgery*, https://doi.org/10.1007/978-3-031-24613-5

**T**



**U**



**V**

MIX
Papier aus verantwortungsvollen Quellen
Paper from responsible sources
FSC® C105338
www.fsc.org

If you have any concerns about our products,
you can contact us on
**ProductSafety@springernature.com**

In case Publisher is established outside the EU,
the EU authorized representative is:
**Springer Nature Customer Service Center GmbH**
**Europaplatz 3, 69115 Heidelberg, Germany**

Printed by Libri Plureos GmbH
in Hamburg, Germany